Boost Your Fertility and Get Pregnant Easily

…Includes How to Take Care of Your Reproductive System, Use of Aphrodisiacs, Herbs, Vitamins and Answers to over 80 Most Frequently Asked Questions Ever, in Fertility and Gynaecology.

Joel O. Akande

Fertility Specialist and Gynaecologist
Founder and Chief Executive Officer at
The Fertility & Gynaecology Centre.

Galaxy Books: Unit of Strategic Insight Publishing (SIP)
Part of Strategic Insight

First published by Strategic Insight Publishing
ISBN 13: 978-1-908064-37-0

British Library Cataloguing in Publication Data
A record for this book is available from the British Library

TABLE OF CONTENTS

Acknowledgement.

I am grateful to God who gives me the strength and knowledge to write. Many thanks to the numerous patients from whom I have learnt over all these years in the course of my clinical practice. My patients have been my textbooks. In the course of writing this book, I have looked at the work of others before me. I may never know the origin of every one of the works but I am grateful.

Dedication

To all long-suffering individuals and couples who with so much determination, endure the indignities of the fertility journey.

Boost Your Fertility

First Things First

It is important that you grasp the meaning of the following terms before you read this book. I recommend you do. I will explain any new term that is not listed here in the respective part of the book when it may first be mentioned.

Amenorrhoea: Stoppage or cessation of periods for over 6 months.

Andrology: The branch of knowledge that deals with the study and treatment of diseases of the male reproductive system.

Anti-oxidants: Antidotes to an internally generated harmful chemical that attack our body organs**.**

Aphrodisiacs: Herb / drug or any sex performance enhancer.

ART: Artificial/Assisted Reproductive Technology.

Assisted Conception: Unnatural conception.

Atrophy: Part of the body that dies off or gradually stops working and dies and wears off.

Azoospermia: No sperm in semen.

Cancer: A dangerous or deadly growth in the body

Conception: The act of getting pregnant.

Chromosomes: They contain and carry genes.

Diabetes Mellitus: Disease of excess and uncontrolled sugar in the blood.

Embryo: The resulting entity following union of egg and sperm.

Endometriosis: Period flow and growth in wrong places and in different parts of the body.

Erectile Dysfunction: Diseases of erection in male.

Fallopian Tube: The tube attached to the womb that transports the sperm, egg and embryo.

Fertilisation: The union of egg and sperm

Fertility: The ability or potential by a woman or man to bear children. Infertility is the opposite.

Fertility Physician /Specialist: Medical doctor who has skills in the science and art of human fertility and reproduction. Fertility doctors offer assessment and treatment of fertility disorders.

Fertility Treatment: Any psychological, medical or surgical intervention that improves fertility in women or men.

Foetus/Fetus: The growing baby in the womb

Follicle: The shell containing the female egg in the ovary.

FSH. Follicle Stimulating Hormone. The brain hormone that controls the growth of eggs in the ovary and sperm in men to grow and mature.

Gametes: The most vital of reproductive cells. They are the eggs and sperms.

Gene: Part of human beings in our cells that carry messages from one generation to the next and instruct our very existence.

Genetics: Relating to genes or the study of genes.

Genotype: The type of gene you carry say sickle cell.

Gynaecology: The branch of knowledge that deals with the study and treatment of diseases of the female reproductive system.

Hereditary, Familial or Inherited disease: Diseases transferred from one generation to the next or specifically within a family.

Hormones: Chemicals that regulate fertility and reproduction and other human functions.

Implantation: The attachment of the embryo to the womb in early baby development.

Inflammation: A medical condition that comes with body injury, swelling, pain and change of colour.

IUI. Intrauterine Insemination (either with the husband's sperm or donor's sperm). Sperm is injected into the woman's uterus around ovulation. Fertilisation is inside the woman.

IVF. In-vitro fertilization (and its variants). A procedure to achieve fertilisation outside the human body. Often used when fallopian tubes are blocked or egg donor is required. It's the most controversial and most expensive of fertility treatments.

LH. Luteinising Hormone: The brain hormone controls the growth of eggs in the ovary. In men, LH causes sperm to grow.

Menopause: Complete stoppage of periods or menstruation at about age of 45 to 52years.

Menstruation: "Periods" consisting of blood and womb debris experienced by women in a cycle.

Oligospermia: Low sperm count (Poor sperm quality)

Oligomenorrhoea: Stoppage or cessation of periods for less than 6 months but more than 35 days.

Ovulation: The release of an egg by the ovary under the influence of LH hormone.

Oxidants: A form of harmful internally generated chemicals that attack our body to cause organ stress (oxidative stress).

PCOS: Polycystic Ovarian Syndrome. A type of disease that causes hormone imbalance.

Pelvis: That human part below the navel that houses the human reproductive system.

Personality Disorder: With or without mental health issue, a weird, odd person with unreasonable behaviour.

PID: Pelvic Inflammatory Disease. Infection of the pelvic organs. The term is applicable to women.

Polyp: Innocent growth that often occurs in the womb or neck of the womb.

Premature menopause: A type of disease leading to complete cessation of periods or menstruation before the age of 45.

Prolactin: A hormone of the brain largely responsible for milk production in the breast.

Psychosis: A form of severe mental illness.

Semen: The combination of sperm, water, sugar and other minerals.

Sperm (male gamete): The key male reproductive element that unites with female egg for fertilisation.

Schizophrenia: A form of severe mental illness.

TTC: Trying to conceive.

Toxins: Unfriendly contamination causing harm to humans.

Vitamins and Supplements: Food additives necessary for normal function of our body but that are made artificially.

Section 1
The Normal Fertility and Reproductive System
"My one purpose in life is to serve as a warning to others."
---Jamie Zawinski

Chapter 1
Before Your Parents Met

It may surprise you if I say that your grandparents living or dead and your great, great, great grandparents who are long dead are still with you. They are in you and living with you. They influenced how you look to some extent, how you behave and what is in you.

You may not have met them, seen, or even heard about them but you are in connection with them.

For a start, all of us human beings, male and female and by any other classification, originally came from the same set of parents. Over time we all went our different ways and inter-married.

We formed different races or somehow, we became different races by reason of colour of our skin, how we look and where we occupy on earth. Indeed, you already know by now that we occupy different regions of the world. That does not remove the simple fact that we originated from one source at the beginning.

Those parents who gave birth to your ancestors continue to pass into the next generation, what scientists call *hereditary (genetic) materials* that are themselves carried by *chromosomes* placed in each of the billions of our individual cells. These genetic materials are coded information that formed our being including the way you look, the way you behave and some effects on your fertility and reproductive systems. Combined with your opposite sexual partner, you will in turn pass your own current inborn material into your own children and children's children and so the life journey continues.

These genetic materials and chromosomes may contain both good or bad items and messages. Example: A certain class of

11

low sperm count may be inherited: genetically passed from fathers to sons. Individuals and family members may inherit some forms of breast cancer or cancer of the ovaries from their parents who had inherited it from their great grandparents.

On the good side, physical appearance, brilliance, arts, literary abilities and even some human conducts may pass on from one generation to the next. Have you ever wondered why a girl or a son looks like a certain member of the family?

Thus, the genetic materials that were passed to you by your ancestral lineage may in part explain your current look and your current conditions. After all, as the saying goes, you do not choose your parents: you take what you inherit.

This is what I meant by your ancestors are still with you.

You just cannot shake them off and you cannot change your ancestors. If you have had good genetic materials passed onto you, under good circumstances, which we shall explain later, chances are that you will turn out well on the condition that you have not behaved in such a way as to damage those genetic materials or potentials.

Therefore, one can safely say that on your part you determine largely what your future children may look like in health and disease. This is the same way that what you are today is a combination of what you received from your parents (good or bad genes, infections, antibodies); the outcome of your own current or past behaviour (infections, drugs, substances, sleep habits, diet); and the effect of the environment (pollution and toxins) that you live in. All of these affect your fertility and reproductive systems as well as having effects on the children that may come through you.

What this ultimately means is that you should choose your partner carefully at least for your own peace and for the benefit of your children. You should conduct yourself carefully too so that you do not damage your potentials and the potentials of your would-be children.

Do not judge a book by its cover. Being hulky, handsome, or being beautiful or pretty may not translate into beneficial fertility status. Why would you want to go through the stress when you can have the certainty before marital commitment in a relationship?

You can also determine your fertility status even after commitment. Why would you pay the price of ignorance or pay for someone else's recklessness? The examples below are put here to make illustrations. You have the liberty to make the choices you will live with.

Example 1.

I once had a man who has had his fertility assessed by my former lecturers while I was still in Medical School over 3 decades ago. I never knew him then. He was diagnosed as azoospermic, (no sperm).

By chance or if you like, by destiny, over thirty years after my graduation from medical school, he came to see me in my own fertility clinic with a wife half his age. He brought the test reports that my teachers had done for him over 30 years ago. I was surprised to see those reports. The wife never knew he had no sperm.

Following our latest assessments, a repeated test confirmed the earlier reports of no sperm. I then had the difficult task of breaking the news to the couple. The young woman was distraught and felt cheated. Lesson: Screen your partner prior to making a commitment.

Example 2.
A couple came to see me for fertility treatment. The wife had HIV (Human Immunodeficiency Virus) infection before the wedding but she did not tell her husband about this infection. He probably did not ask either. The discovery was made in our clinic that she was infected. You can guess the pain and surprise that clouded the room when we discussed the issue. Lesson: Screen your partner before you have sex. Your decision will affect your children.

Example 3.
A couple mistakenly believed that each of them had AA genotype before wedding and went to marry. The first child resulted in sickle cell child and a life burden for the couple. Lesson: Know your genetic status and that of your partner before you get serious. Your decision will affect your children.

Example 4.
A couple were in marriage and produced 5 children. The mother had a mental health breakdown before she married. All of her children developed one form of schizophrenia or other psychotic illnesses. These were clearly mental health illnesses that had been passed on from one generation to another. Lesson: You are in position to determine the fate of your children to some extent. Do it.

Example 5.
In another case, a young newly wedded couple came to see me for fertility treatment. It turned out that the man knew before the couple's wedding that he was suffering from erectile dysfunction ('impotence" or inability to sustain erection for the purpose of having sex or long standing failure of erection, to be precise). Yet he went ahead to marry this beautiful bride.

Of course, the frustration and sense of loss were visible on the wife's face when she discovered the husband's hidden challenges. Lesson: Know yourself and your partner through and through before you get too far. Avoid the tears and the pain of infertility. The choice is yours.

Boost Your Fertility

Chapter 2
How Your Reproductive System Works.

If your trying to conceive (TTC) journey is to be meaningful and if you are to be part of the solution to your fertility challenges, you need to understand how your body and reproductive system work. As this book is about education and empowerment, let me inform you now that fertility consists of three parts. Not arranged in any particular order of importance, the first is gynaecology which deals with functions, structure and treatment of diseases of female reproductive systems. The second is andrology which concerns the functions, structure, and treatment of diseases of male reproductive systems. The third is fertility which deals with coming together of both gynaecology and andrology. That is, if a person desires (note the very crucial word "desires") to have a child or reproduce, he or she uses her reproductive system along with the willing opposite gender to achieve this purpose of conception and childbearing.

Fertility therefore is all about *desire and choice* to reproduce. You may have a perfect reproductive system and you have no desire or intention to reproduce. In that case, you do not have issues with fertility (or infertility).

That said, let us take a look at the human reproductive system.

The Female Reproductive System
Functions:
The ovaries
There two ovaries one on each side of your body and each ovary contains eggs. In each menstrual cycle, about 10-15 eggs will develop in either of the ovaries. Which one of the ovaries will produce these eggs in each month is a matter of random selection. One of the developing eggs will dominate

the others. This leader among the developing eggs will be the one to be released. This process of release of an egg is called *ovulation.*

The rest of the eggs will die. The developing eggs or follicles produce the female hormone oestrogen and progesterone. The follicle is the shell with the egg inside it.

Together, these hormones shape the life of women and conception. However, the ovary and the hormones are controlled from the brain with another set of hormones called FSH and LH (Follicle Stimulating Hormone and Luteinising Hormone)). For balance, it may interest you that the female also produces a little of the male hormone called testosterone.

Female Reproductive System

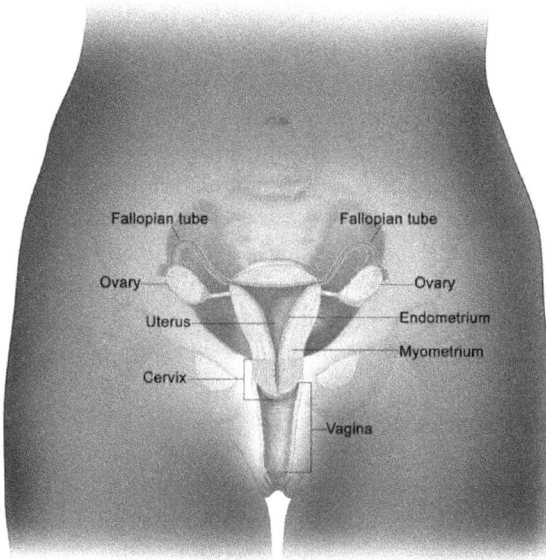

Credit and Copyright: National Cancer Institute

18

Fallopian Tubes

The purpose of the Fallopian tube, one on each side of the female body, is to allow eggs and sperms to pass and to meet each other for the purposes of fertilisation to form an embryo which is the new baby. Once fertilisation takes place, the fallopian tube allows the passage of the new baby into the uterus (womb).

The uterus

The work of the uterus is to receive, house and nourish the new developing baby(embryo). Once the embryo lands and starts attaching (this process of attaching to the womb is called implantation), the womb or uterus has the function to nourish, keep safe and sustain the growing baby until the time of delivery.

The uterus serves other functions: it allows the sperm to pass from the vagina into the uterus through the fallopian tube on the way to meeting the egg for fertilisation.

Finally, the uterus allows the womb lining (which we often refer to as endometrium) and products of menstruation to flow outside the body during menstruation also commonly called "period".

The cervix (The neck of the womb)

The cervix serves to control what goes in and out of the uterus. In performing this duty, the cervix can produce friendly cervical mucus during ovulation that allows sperm to flow in. Also, the cervix can relax to allow babies to be born. In similar manner, the cervix can relax to allow products of menstruation to flow out. I want you to take note of the words "cervical mucus" because it has a larger than life role to play in fertility. Unfriendly cervical mucus may kill the sperm or not allow the sperm to pass through to the womb on the way

19

to meeting the egg as earlier mentioned. This is one of the causes of infertility.

The vagina

The vagina has the duty of receiving the penis during sexual intercourse and to allow sperm to be deposited in its space. It produces a liquid that allows sex to be enjoyed. This liquid helps in what is commonly called "getting wet" during sex. The vaginal environment is warm and friendly for the survival of sperm. Another very important function of the vagina is to allow babies to pass through it into the world. Similarly, it provides a pathway for products of menstruation to pass to the outside world.

It's important to note that the vagina has its own self-cleaning and self-maintaining bacteria. Except if disease sets in, you don't have to help the vagina in its sacred duty of self-cleaning.

The vulva

The vulva is what you see when you look at the female reproductive system from outside. At the top end of the vulva is the clitoris and a short distance from the clitoris underneath is the urethra whereby urine ("wee" or "pee" or "water") flows out. Apart from housing these important organs, the vulva is a structure of beauty and making of necessary products to maintain a sexual appeal.

One other important function of the vulva and surrounding muscles is that together, they control what goes in and out of the vagina. In doing this job, the vulva provides grip and firmness for the penis during sex.

A word on menstruation

Menstruation (or Period) is a flow of womb lining (endometrium) along with blood and other tissues from the womb.

Period is a message. Period is telling the person that in the cycle "A" that just ended, the woman was not pregnant. As a result, the womb lining that was prepared to receive an embryo was cleared out to make way for a new cycle and new preparation for likely embryo in this new cycle "B". Menstruation is just the outflow of womb lining at the end of each cycle if pregnancy did not occur. The amount of blood flow in the entire "*period*" time varies and may be about 4 tablespoons to 8 tablespoons. Period can sometimes last up to 7 days. The usual range is 3 to 5 days. It may be painful in persons who are young and have never conceived. In others, infection and pelvic diseases may cause the pain. Heavy period flow is a disease and may be due to either fibroid or an under-performing thyroid. Period is not the same thing as miscarriage or threatening miscarriage. Bleeding in early pregnancy may also come from the gripping of the embryo on the womb. This is what we refer to as implantation haemorrhage.

The Male Reproductive System

The testes
The testes are two "balls" placed in the scrotal sac that hangs out between the thighs. It's the equivalent of ovaries found in women. The main purpose is to produce sperms at a temperature of about 32-34°C. Sperm is a major part of semen. Semen is what we see when a man ejaculates (releases sperm). Therefore, you should not confuse sperm with semen. Remember that the human body temperature is about 36.2 to 37.6C. Therefore, the making of sperm takes place outside the main body at a cooler temperature.

Male Reproductive System

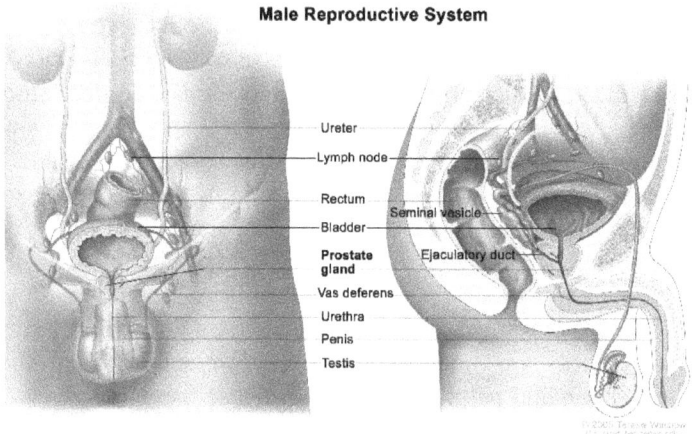

Ureter
Lymph node
Rectum
Seminal vesicle
Bladder
Prostate gland
Ejaculatory duct
Vas deferens
Urethra
Penis
Testis

Credit and Copyright: National Cancer Institute

The second function of the testes is to produce testosterone. Testosterone is the male hormone. There are other hormones that the testes produce). For balance, it may interest you that the male also produces a little of the female hormone called estradiol and progesterone.

The epidydimis (the male tube)
The main function of this organ is in part to store the sperm and when required carry or allow the sperm to pass from the store towards the penis and into the female vagina during sex.

Prostate
The prostate's major role is to add sugar (fructose), liquid, zinc and other nutrients on to the sperm coming from the epidydimis to form semen. It also has a control gateway that

allows sperm to pass during sex or urine to pass when empty-ing the bladder. Except in disease, urine and sperm do not mix.

The urethra
The urethra is the final pathway for either the urine or semen to pass to the outside world. From the urinary bladder the ure-thra passes through the penis outward.

The penis
The function of the penis is to allow urine to pass when we empty our bladder. In terms of fertility, the penis is the natural organ to deposit sperm or semen in the vagina of the female. The penis has no other function.

A word on "wet dreams"
The closest event to menstruation as it happens in women, is wet dreams in men and boys. This wet dream is the sudden release of semen especially during sleep. Sex dreams are com-mon in men. This event should not cause alarm if a boy or a man bed wets with semen. It's a natural way of clearing the sperm store.

In both men and women:
The brain
The ultimate control of our reproductive system rests with the brain. The brain through an organ that goes by a name, pitui-tary, sends signals to either ovaries or testes to produce eggs (women) or sperm(men) as the case may be. The thyroid and adrenal glands are other organs that help in the control of our fertility.

The breast

The breast is part of our fertility and reproductive system especially in women. Events in the breast may disturb your fertility. If the breast is discharging milky or other coloured substances, it may indicate that there is an underlying problem with your hormones and conception could become difficult. Diseases of the breast could have links elsewhere in the reproductive system such as the thyroid, ovaries and the brain.

In summary, we must protect all these reproductive structures from damage. Our behaviours and how we use our body in general and our reproductive system in particular could affect our health and our ability to bear children. We will further explain in the next chapters, conditions that may damage our reproductive system and cause us conception difficulties.

Chapter 3
The Ticking Fertility Clock.

Once a spark of life is kindled in the womb or in assisted conception, which takes place outside the human body, the life clock for the individual starts to run. Ironically, death also starts to run at the same time.

Take note of these facts as written below. Read this page again if necessary to grasp these key points. These details form the bedrock of human fertility.

The Female Fertility Clock.
While still in the womb, a female baby fertility clock begins to run from the age of about 4 months counting from the meeting of sperm and egg (fertilisation). At the age of 4 months or so, the female baby has the highest number of eggs that is ever possible. At this age, the egg count ranges from 6 to 7 million eggs in both ovaries.

At birth, the 7 million eggs will have diminished to about 2 million at best. They simply die off.

At about the time of the first period of the female person, which may be anytime between 11 to 15 years, the 2 million eggs have further decreased to 500,000.

This reduction of eggs available for conception continues as the female individual advances in age.

By the time the woman lives up to the age of 37 years, the total number of eggs available will be in the range of 25,000. From age of 35 years and beyond, the death and reduction of the number of eggs will begin to diminish at a faster rate than before. Thus, by the age of 50, the total number of eggs available for possible conception has fallen from 7 million while in the womb to a mere 1000 at the age of 50 years.

Quality versus quantity
Just as the number or quantity of eggs is getting smaller by age, so is the quality. Just as we age physically in our world, so do the eggs. Therefore, amongst the fertility factors to consider, age is at the very top of the pyramid. The poor quality in female eggs may result in a disabled child or an increase in miscarriages. For a fact, fertility diminishes with age.

Aging of eggs at ovulation
When an egg is released at ovulation, such an egg has 24 hours to live. If not fertilised, the egg will die. To be sure, the first 12 to 18 hours following ovulation is crucial to success if conception is to occur. If the fertilised egg is choked by an unfriendly environment, it will die.

Male Fertility Clock
Unlike the female, the male does not have similar fertility clock. In general, a typical male may continue to fertilise an egg well into old age.

The sperm cycle:
Similar to the female, men have their own cycles. It takes about 84 days to form sperm and an additional 10 to 15 days for maturation: this gives a total of about 100 days for sperm to be produced and matured. By the time the sperm is released, additional minerals and nutrients are added along the way while in the male reproductive system to provide the energy that the sperm will need to reach the egg waiting for it in the female reproductive system.

Stamina
However, the stamina of a typical man begins to increase as he advances in age which would be at puberty from say 15

years old. Men's sexual and physical stamina starts to decrease from about the age of 40 and beyond.

By age of 65, the quality of the semen and sperm start to show flaws. This poor quality in sperm, just as in females, may also result in a disabled child and increased miscarriages. Example of such disability is autism. As men age, so does their sexual stamina.

Clocking of sperm in female reproductive system.

Under normal conditions free of any complication, the sperm can live 3 to 5 or even 7 days in the reproductive system of a female. This is especially so if the female is healthy and her reproductive system is not hostile to the sperms.

Timing and Time in Fertility

Nearly everything in the world of fertility relates to time. Timing is indeed everything in fertility. From ovulation (14 days before the first day of your next period) and fertilisation (must happen within 24 hours of ovulation); the duration of the movement of an embryo to the womb from the fallopian tube (takes about 3-5 days), to the time of implantation to the duration of pregnancy (40weeks) and the delivery date are all timed. Remember this, especially if you plan to conceive naturally.

Chapter 4
Care for Your Reproductive System.

Our reproductive system deserves our respect. You should consider your fertility pathway as sacred and be protected from damage if we are to achieve our aim of reproducing our kind. The next section of the book offers you little steps you can take to boost your fertility and take care of your reproductive system.

Nutrition
Our reproductive system is an essential part of our body. If you are missing in maintaining the right balance of foods and water, your fertility and overall health may suffer. Eat good food consisting of leaves, vegetables, proteins, carbohydrates (starch), vitamins, minerals, fat and water: all in the right balance. At the same time, avoid processed food as much as possible. Natural food is much better.

Tidiness
Keep your reproductive system tidy. In general, keep your body tidy and free of contamination such as toxins and infections. Look after the surrounding and overlaying skin areas. Keep the internal organs active and free from infections or toxic substances.

Right temperature and humidity.
In both men and women, our body needs to be kept within certain temperature range not higher than 37.6C and not lower than 32C.

For men:
The production of sperm takes place at about 32C to 34 Celsius. Higher temperature generated by computers, tight pants, leg crossing, long distance driving, long bicycle ride, long night TV watching, mobile phones in the pocket and hot water baths, may badly affect the production of sperm.

For women:
High humidity and raised temperature may affect the health of the skin around the vulva and vagina. Such high humidity may cause thrush or yeast and bacteria to grow in the vulva and vagina. Vulva, vagina and pelvis generally need good ventilation to maintain health and prevent diseases.

Exercises and weight: Good health and indeed reproductive health and fertility health need regular and focused physical exercises. The breast needs movements and touching. The body fat and weight need to be put in reasonable range of health in what is measured as BMI (Body-Mass-Index) that is appropriate for the person's height.

Being underweight or overweight and obese may lead to difficulties to conceive. What is the ideal weight? To do this, measure your height in meters and your weight in kilograms. Then calculate your Body-Mass-Index (BMI).

BMI = Weight (Kg) $\div$ (Height)^2. Your ideal weight should be between 18 to 24.9. If your BMI is between 25 and 30, you are overweight. If you are over 30, you are obese.

Physical exercises help to reduce body fat, and blood sugar levels. Physical exercises help us to eliminate toxins from our body.

Regular exercises help maintain good hormone levels and improve fertility. In women, exercises lower estradiol levels which is a good thing for overall health and reproduction.

High estradiol is associated with fibroid, endometrial cancer, breast cancer and infertility. In men, exercises increase testosterone levels, which is good for sperm production and sexual stamina. Exercising should be moderate and not more than 150 minutes per week for both men and women. Keep your BMI between 18 and 25 values.

Stress and worrying.
Keep your stress level down. Stress increases stress hormones called cortisol and adrenalin. Under stress, the body is tensed-up and hormones become chaotic. If you are stressed or worrying, you may start missing your periods or have scanty periods. Ovulation may become erratic and achieving conception gets difficult. The urge to have sex becomes low and uninteresting. The body tires easily. You age faster with stress. In addition, for men the urge to have sex is low and sustaining an erection becomes a challenge.

Sleep
Endeavour to sleep well. As an adult, you need a minimum of 5 hours sleep per 24 hours. If you can, achieve this sleep pattern at night. Night sleep is just natural but it may not be so for everyone. Go to bed at about the same time every night. Be consistent. Poor sleep, may generate anxiety, tiredness and depression. Poor sleep produces irritation and anger. The brain cannot function optimally when you sleep poorly. As a result, the hormones are imbalanced, chaotic or unpredictable. You become stressed. Ovulation may not happen and getting pregnant becomes a distant hope.

Toxins
Toxins are everywhere. They are found in water, air, food, food packaging, industrial wastes, cosmetics, hair spray, body

spray, cooking ware and pesticides. Do your study well. Read the content and sources before using that food and non-food products. Pollutants are enemies to our health and fertility. Use glass to store water for drinking and china for heating in microwave. Further, infections may produce toxins and other damages, which can last longer than after the infection has been taken care of. Together, toxins damage our general health and fertility.

Chapter 5
How to Achieve Conception Naturally.

To start with, conception is a natural event. When pregnancy does not happen, it means something went wrong in the reproductive system of the male, female, or both, as mentioned earlier. How then should one conduct oneself to get pregnant naturally?

Female:

The starting point is that you should know how to calculate your menstrual cycle. You should also know the symptoms of ovulation. Let me repeat what I said in the last chapter. Menstrual period is a signal that in this cycle, you did not get pregnant. The count of a cycle starts from the first day of menstruation and ends on the day before the first day of the next cycle. The normal cycles range from 21 days for some women and up to 35 days for others. Most women will fall anything in between these extremes. Many women will have a 28-day cycle. The rule of thumb is that ovulation will occur 14 days before the first day of your cycle.

Therefore, if you have a 28- day cycle, your ovulation is likely to be on day 14. For 35-day cycle, your ovulation is likely to be around the 21st day of your cycle. If you have 21-day cycle, you are likely to ovulate on day 7. If you have a 30-day cycle, your ovulation day will fall on day 16 of your cycle.

Symptoms of ovulation include a rise in your body temperature by about 0.2Celcius to 0.5Celcius. That is, after ovulation, average basal body temperature increases to between 97.6°F (36.4°C) and 98.6°F (37°C). You might have heaviness and fullness in your breast with some discomfort around the nipple. You may also have increased urge for sex. In the vagina, a clear stretchy jelly-like discharge (cervical mucus), under the influence of progesterone (female hormone) indicates ovulation has occurred.

To determine your menstrual cycle length and ovulation date, you need to keep a diary of your symptoms, temperature and experiences over a 3 to 6-month period.

Sex

For you to get pregnant naturally, start having sex 2 days before your ovulation and continue up to three days after your ovulation. Repeat this in the next cycle until you get pregnant. Getting pregnant naturally, requires that you have a lot of sex. You can do this daily or on alternative days.

There is evidence that even ordinarily, if you have sex 2 to 3 times in a week not minding ovulation day, you have a good chance of getting pregnant.

Naturally, it may interest you that sperm can live in the female reproductive system for up to 5 days. This may not happen if the cervical mucus is hostile to the sperm, there is a blockage at the cervix, the womb and tubes are blocked or there is an infection. The sperm may also not live longer if the sperm is itself weak or deformed.

A female egg released during ovulation, will only live for 24 hours with its strength and quality diminishing by the hour. The first 12 to 18 hours after ovulation represent the optimal time for the sperm to fertilise the egg. This knowledge of sperm and egg life longevity is very important to achieving pregnancy naturally. Timing is everything in fertility.

The conduct of sex.

Vaginal sex with orgasm is better and the contraction movements of the vagina, cervix and the womb tend to suck in the sperm towards the egg. I say vaginal sex because oral sex or sex by any other means, will not lead to conception.

For the female, to avoid sperm backflow or leakage, lay on your back. Support your bottom with a pillow to elevate the vagina. Stay in bed. Raise your leg up or put it against the wall for a while.

For the *male,* ensure the vagina receives the semen and all of it and in as many sexual rounds as possible.

Enhance your potential to conceive naturally (men and women alike).
Pregnancy may not survive in a hostile physical or mental health environment. Therefore, make sure you remove barriers that may work against sustaining a pregnancy.

Doing the following will help. *Eat balanced and nutritious food.* In particular, food that contains fruits and vegetables which will supply the vitamins (B, C, E) and minerals that were discussed earlier. Eat fish to help you with omega-3 (DHA).

Avoid the following:
Alcohol, nicotine, cocaine, antimalarials other than chloroquine with chlorpheneramine. Avoid foods, herbs and other drugs that work against pregnancy. Some herbs and foods may terminate an ongoing pregnancy.

Ventilation
Allow your external reproductive areas to receive *ventilation.* You could sleep naked at night to cool down your body temperature and allow ventilation. In the day, wear loose

garments around your reproductive organs for sake of ventilation.

Detoxfication

Finally, remember that some *substances* create barriers against getting pregnant. It may be necessary for you to undergo a period of *detoxification of toxins* from your body.

If you do all of the above recommendations, you have set yourself up for success through natural conception.

Section 2
Fertility Disorders
"I think the one lesson I have learned is that there is no sub-
stitute for paying attention."
---Diane Sawyer

Chapter 6
Common Disorders Causing Infertility

Infertility is the inability to achieve conception after 12 months of trying, without the use of family planning protection. Infertility can result from such simple acts as refusal of partners to have sex. Failure to conceive could result from the absence of one partner. Infertility may also be due to serious physical and mental health abnormalities, which we will now go through.

For Women

Hormone Imbalance is a common umbrella name for disorders of the fertility hormone system (the brain, ovaries in women or testes in men. The thyroid (an organ, covered up by skin, in front of the neck) and adrenals in both women and men). See Section 1 for what is normal reproductive system. Hormone imbalance has several causes. Practically, anything that cause disturbance of the normal functions of the hormones is a cause of such imbalance. Stress, over-exercising, sleeplessness, poor nutrition, medication, family planning hormones and herbs may be responsible. Diseases of the brain (pituitary), underacting or overacting thyroid are common. Polycystic ovarian syndrome (PCOS) may also cause hormone imbalance. PCOS occurs in about 12 to 15% of women and PCOS is well known to cause problems with ovulation, irregular vaginal bleeding, cause poor vaginal lubrication and PCOS is also responsible for some miscarriages.

Lack of ovulation (known as anovulation) is responsible for infertility in a third (30%) of cases in women. This in itself may be due to some causes of hormonal imbalance as mentioned above.

39

Fallopian tubal blockage is a cause of infertility in a third (30%) of women seeking to get pregnant. This condition may be because one or both tubes are blocked. Causes of tubal blockage include infection, previous operations in the pelvic area, endometriosis and fibroid.

Diseases of the womb such as *uterine adhesions* (womb lining and the walls of the womb are stuck together), or *large fibroid* that blocks the tubes and occupy large space in the womb, may cause infertility.

The Cervix may have *growths* that block the movement of sperm. Cervical mucus may be *hostile* and not allowing the sperm to pass to fertilise the eggs as we mentioned before.

The Vagina may lack lubrication (getting wet during sex or in preparation for sex) due to anxiety or hormone imbalance. On the one hand, this may make sex difficult and on the other hand it could cause infertility. Still, without lubrication, the vagina may become hostile to sperm.

The Ovaries may suffer from diseases that prevent it from doing its job well. Examples are PCOS and endometriosis, cancer, radiation and chemotherapy exposures. Endometriosis is a very common and serious disease that occurs in about one in every ten of the general female population; in women with pain, infertility, or both, the rate is one-third (30%) to half (50%) of such population suffering from endometriosis. About a quarter (25%) to half (50%) of infertile women have endometriosis, and one-third (30%) to half of women with endometriosis are infertile. Endometriosis may damage the ovaries or block the tubes.

Mental health issues on their own such as depression (feeling low in mood or spirit lasting over two weeks at a stretch), anxiety(agitation, being restless in mind and body), psychosis and stress may seriously affect your ability to conceive. The medications for treatment of mental illnesses may also produce effects that make it impossible to conceive.

Medical illnesses like diabetes mellitus especially in uncontrolled blood sugar (which sometimes occurs with PCOS), bowel diseases, and liver and kidney illnesses may lead to infertility.

Aging of the individual especially with the ovaries rapidly losing eggs is a major cause of infertility.

Previous surgery or damage to the womb, tubes and cervix may sometimes lead to complications (tubal blockage, weak cervix, uterine adhesions) and infertility.

For Men
Poor semen and sperm are major causes of infertility in men. For our purpose, anything that disturbs the production, the storage and the movement of sperm may seriously affect the sperm functions. The semen contains sperm. The sperm in their millions along with liquid surrounding them is call semen. If the liquid semen is too thick or of bad colour or odour and not releasing the sperm it contains within it *on time*, the sperm may be locked down. The result is infertility as the sperm is unable to move.

Oligospermia or low sperm count (I prefer *poor sperm qualities*) may be due to infection, hostile environment caused by oxidative stress (see our discussion on glutathione under vitamins and supplements).

Oxidative stress may be due to cigarette toxins, drugs, and alcohol. Oxidative stress may be the after-effect of infection. Heating up the testes via tight pants, hot bath, long bicycle rides, long driving hours, laptop, mobile use near testes or placing mobile/cellphones in pockets close to testes, and long hours of watching TV beyond 10pm could all lead to poor sperm qualities. Majorly, abnormal sperm qualities due to heating is due to varicocele. *Varicocele* may require surgery for correction. Varicocele is unwanted large collection of blood vessels within around testes. The blood vessels heat up the testes and cause low sperm count.

Gaps or shortfall in zinc and other nutrients as discussed under *Vitamins and Supplements*, could cause poor sperm qualities.

Another important cause of fertility failure in men *is erectile dysfunction or popularly called impotence*. This is failure to have erection when needed and for a length of time required. Erectile dysfunction also includes releasing the sperm too early (premature ejaculation) and ejaculating too late (delayed ejaculation) as well as ejaculating in the wrong place along the man's reproductive track.

Men suffer from *hormone imbalance* too. Male family planning medicines or surgery could cause infertility issues. High prolactin produces breast discharge in men and is a sign of underlying hormone imbalance. Thyroid illnesses in men could delay conception, just as in women.

Men do suffer from diabetes, liver diseases, kidney illnesses, genetic diseases like sickle cell and cancers. All of these *medical illnesses* may disturb male fertility.

For both men and women, long distance relationships and failure to engage in sex will delay conception.

Infections

Infections generally are threats to our individual and collective health. Infections of the female reproductive tract account for a third (30%) of fertility problems in women. In men, a similar challenge. Such infections are ones that are passed from one person to the other through sex. We call them sexually transmitted infections (STI) and they include gonorrhoea, chlamydia, syphilis, lymphogranuloma venerum, herpes simplex, human papilloma virus (HPV), human immune-deficiency virus (HIV), hepatitis B and C. These infections are not to be taken lightly. Left unattended or delay in getting prompt treatment, they can cause significant damage to your general health, fertility and even cause death of the person affected. Yet other infections are thrush or candida and scabies. Some are not infections classed as STI but once they get into one partner, it may affect the other person. They are called non-STI. The common ones are *staphylococcus aureus, E.coli* and other non-STI infections. Staphylococcus aureus is particularly notorious as it affects billions of people all over the world.

In both male and female, all of these infections may damage the reproductive track or disturb conception in one way or another. Sadly, women by their biological nature, are less likely to show symptoms of infections than men, until things become too complicated.

The author's approach and advice is that you should screen your sexual partner medically before you get into the business of having sexual intercourse. Each person should consider sticking with the other person only. In same thinking, if you have or suspect any symptom such as pain, rash, swelling, sore and discharge in your reproductive system, get checked medically immediately as well as yearly or at 6-monthly intervals whether you have symptoms or not.

Do not be ashamed. Prevention is better than cure. Some of the infections are deadly and may kill you if you allow it to spread or allow it to cause you more damage due to delay in seeking help.
Further, hepatitis B and HPV do have vaccinations. Other vaccines such as for chlamydia are in development and not yet ready for general use.

Chapter 7
Myths, Untruths and Facts About Your Reproductive System

In probably all cultures of the world, people have built myths and folklores to surround the female reproductive system. This book is not about disputing such myths and untruths. This book is about fertility and enhancing both female and male reproductive potentialities. Let us therefore mention a few of the very common practices and beliefs that deserve our attention.

Vagina steaming and "cleaning"

By nature, the female and male reproductive system should be regarded as "sacred" in the sense that these organs should be kept away from contamination (chemical, infection or by any other interference). The more the reproductive system remains free of unnecessary contamination, the higher its potential for fertility.

For a start, the vaginal area has its own "laundry" cleaning system. There are "in-house security" bacteria that cleans and defends the vagina from infection.

Secondly, vagina produces its own chemicals that maintain PH (Potential of Hydrogen) which measures how acidic or alkalinic the vagina is. This vagina PH's duty is to be friendly to the sperms and the health of the reproductive system. It produces some normal secretions, which may appear as a discharge under some conditions. Normally, vagina does not produce discharge of concern.

Therefore, if you introduce heat in the name of steaming or chemicals and objects such as "pearls" that come in various names, you may be damaging the health of your vagina and your fertility potentials.

In addition, you do not need antiseptic soaps or cosmetics to keep the vagina free of bad odour or discharge.

Example:

We once had a woman who was to undergo embryo transfer in an IVF cycle. On the day, she was told not to put on body spray or cosmetics. In spite of the advanced warning, her whole vagina area was perfumed. You can guess the outcome of the procedure.

However, the vagina area, just like the pelvic area of men, needs a lot and frequent ventilation to keep the temperature down. If you allow your pelvis to become humid or hot and moist by any means, such an environment may lead to bacterial infection and growth of yeasts (thrush or candidiasis).

"I am 43 years old. I am still having my period, so I am still fertile and able to conceive."

There is no truth in this at all. Menstruation is not equal to fertility. In fact, true menstruation is a message that tells you that "in this cycle, you have not been pregnant, sorry."

In addition, we do know that there is what is called *anovulatory* cycle. That means a cycle with menstruation but no ovulation.

Furthermore, with increasing early menopause in women in modern times, and premature ovarian dysfunction rising, the ovaries may fail even though you have periods occasionally.

In addition, there are many drugs and herbs out there, that may artificially cause you to have "menstruation" even in absence of ovulation. Without ovulation, we cannot talk of fertility except physicians intervene artificially.

"I am still young, so time is on my side to conceive."

Age is important in fertility. As we pointed out earlier, peak female fertility is 22 to 32 years but fertility can be extended to much later than 32 years and earlier than 22years. However, for various reasons, age is not the only measure of fertility. Errors in life or during pregnancy may affect fertility. Therefore, you cannot solely, rely on your age as a measure of your fertility.

"My ovulation is on the 14th day of my cycle or my mid-cycle."
Menstrual period is a signal that in this cycle, you did not get pregnant. The count of a cycle starts from the first day of menstruation and ends on the day before the first day of the next cycle. Normal cycles range from 21 days for some women and up to 35 days for others. Most women will fall anything in-between these extremes. Many women will have a 28-day cycle. The rule of the thumb is that ovulation will occur approximately 14 days before the first day of your next period. Therefore, if you have a 28-day cycle, your ovulation is likely to be on day 14. For 35-day cycle, your ovulation is likely to be around the 21st day of your cycle. If you have 21-day cycle, you are likely to ovulate on the 7th day. If you have a 30-day cycle, your ovulation day will fall on day 16th of your cycle.

"I am not pregnant because of sperm leakage after sex."
To start with, semen is what a man releases during sex, presumably inside the vagina. Semen contains millions of sperm. The minimum sperm required to work for fertilization is twenty million. Ordinarily, at ejaculation during sex, released semen which maximum volume is under 5mls (teaspoon) is like a jelly. It must become liquefied (within one hour) soon after discharge to release the tiny and vulnerable sperms.
Most pregnancies result from just one sperm that got to the egg first most efficiently. Of the millions of sperms released,

only about 200 will get to the egg for the purpose of fertilisation. Of these, the first successful sperm that gains entry into the egg is the winner. The rest of the sperm will die along the way. You need just a little semen to fire the successful group sperms. The rest of semen and sperm that did not move forward for fertilisation may leak out of the vagina or the liquid will get absorbed through the vaginal walls into the body.

Therefore, it's not true that leakage of sperm contributes to infertility.

Even assuming that sperm leakage is true cause of infertility, to help sperm migration towards the egg, you can stay in bed after sex, or you use pillow to support your bottom or raise your legs against the wall during sex.

In some cases, sperm leakage may be due to growths in the neck of the womb (cervix), uterine adhesion, absent cervix or uterus, big fibroids, hostile cervical mucus and when the penis is poorly inserted into vagina during sex. If you are concerned about sperm leakage, you should see a fertility physician or a gynaecologist for examination.

Circumcision

Circumcision of the female is very concerning; the practice is based on the false belief that circumcision reduces the female sexual urge. On the contrary, in part, irrespective of the degree and extent, circumcision damages the female reproductive system and leaves a psychological injury in the body and mind of the victim. Circumcision may make vaginal delivery difficult. It may also make sex less pleasurable and the female is denied a major biological joy.

Boost Your Fertility

Section 3.
Solutions to Fertility Disorders & Fertility Boosting.

"I think the one lesson I have learned is that there is no substitute for paying attention."
---Diane Sawyer

Chapter 8
Vitamins, Supplements and Fertility.

Warning: You should seek the support of a qualified medical practitioner before you use vitamins and supplements.

Good food and balanced diet are essential for fertility. The absence of minerals and vitamins in our food may make our ability to conceive difficult. Herbs and drugs influence the character and direction of our fertility. Mentioned next are key minerals, vitamins and herbs that affect fertility. The following are the fertility boosters you may consider to help you.

Vitamins:
Vitamin A (Retinol)
Vitamin A works to help us maintain good eyesight. The vitamin also helps to maintain growth and the soundness of cells including reproductive cells. Vitamin A is essential for the maintenance of the male reproductive tract, sperm development and storage. In the female, vitamin A is important in the stages of egg development and baby in the womb (fetus) growth.

Where to find Vitamin A: Vitamin A is almost exclusively in animal products, such as human milk, glandular meats, liver and fish liver oils (especially), egg yolk, and whole milk and dairy products. Vitamin A is also used to fortify processed foods that may include sugar, cereals, condiments, fats, and oils. Vitamin A are found in green leafy vegetables (e.g., spinach, amaranth, and young leaves from various sources), yellow vegetables (e.g., pumpkins, squash, and carrots), and yellow and orange non-citrus fruits (e.g., mangoes, apricots, and papaya). Red palm oil produced in several countries worldwide is especially rich in vitamin A.

Vitamin B1(Thiamin)
Vitamin B1 plays an important role in the development of good quality eggs in women.
Where to find B1: food sources of thiamine include beef, liver, dried milk, nuts, oats, oranges, pork, eggs, seeds, legumes, peas and yeast. Foods are also fortified with thiamine. Some foods that are often fortified with B1 are rice, pasta, breads, cereals and flour.

Vitamin B2(Riboflavin)
Pregnancy demands higher riboflavin intake as it crosses the placenta(after-birth of baby organ). It helps quality development of the growing babies.
Where to find B2: Foods that are particularly rich in riboflavin include eggs, organ meats (kidneys and liver), lean meats, and milk. Green vegetables also contain riboflavin.
Because riboflavin is soluble in water, about twice as much riboflavin content is lost in cooking water when foods are boiled as when they are prepared in other ways, such as by steaming or microwaving.

Vitamin B3(Niacin)
This vitamin is an anti-oxidant (see explanation of antioxidant under glutathione and in First Thing First) and helps maintain the integrity of the cells: both eggs and sperms. Lack of B3 may lead to impotence in men and dysmenorrhea (painful periods) in women.
Where to find Niacin: niacin sources include red meat, fish, poultry, fortified breads and cereals, and enriched pasta and peanuts.

Vitamin B6.
B6 plays more of a role during pregnancy than pre-pregnancy but it should form part of overall vitamin intake balance. Vitamin B6 also plays a role in brain development of babies.
Where to find B6: pork, poultry, such as chicken or turkey, some fish peanuts soya beans, wheat germ, oats and bananas.

Vitamin B7 (Biotin or vitamin H)
B7 is crucial for maintaining reproductive functions and normal embryo growth. Biotin can act as a promising sperm motility enhancer. Biotin can boost sperm motility and prolong the existence sperms that are frozen for IVF/IUI. Studies have shown that deficiency of biotin during the pregnancy period leads to abnormal baby development.
Where to find biotin: egg yolk, organ meats (liver, kidney), nuts, like almonds, peanuts, pecans, and walnuts, nut butters, soybeans and other legumes, whole grains and cereals, cauliflower, bananas.

Myo-inositol/Inositol ("Vitamin B8")
Note: myo-inositol or its sister mirror image inositol is not a vitamin. In a PCOS, B8 would relate to an improvement in insulin sensitivity and as a result, increased glucose uptake into the cells. Evidence suggests that treatment with myo-inositol in women with PCOS results in better fertilization rates and a clear trend to a better embryo quality.
Where to find myoinositol: fruits, beans, grains, and nuts. Cantaloupe, oats, bran, and citrus fruits (other than lemons) are especially rich in myo-inositol. Cooking or freezing fruits and vegetables reduces their inositol content.

Vitamin B9 (Folic Acid and folate):
Folic acid is an artificial drug—the tablet you take. Folate is the one that occurs naturally in food. Folic acid will still have to be converted before becoming useful in the body.

Folate affects function of the ovaries, implantation of embryo and the entire process of pregnancy. Folate is essential for sperm development. Lack of folic acid in a pregnant woman may cause spinal bifida(a diseases of the backbone) in the newborn.

Where to find folate: Liver, fresh green vegetables. Leafy green vegetables, like spinach, broccoli, and lettuce, orange juice, fish, chicken breast, beans, peas, and lentils. Fruits like lemons, bananas, and melons. Fortified and enriched products, like some breads, juices, and cereals.

Vitamin B12
B12 acts by increasing sperm count, and by enhancing sperm motility and reducing sperm DNA damage.

Where to find B12: Products from plant-eating animals such as milk, meat, and eggs.

Vitamin C (Ascorbic Acid).
Vitamin C: plays key role in hormone production in both male and females, and its ability to protect cells from oxidants (or free radicals) which we mentioned earlier. Free radicals are damaging to cells during their development. Vitamin C is important during fertilization. Vitamin C is an anti-oxidant.

Where to find Vitamin C: Fruits and vegetables are the best sources of vitamin C. Citrus fruits, red pepper, tomatoes and tomato juice, and potatoes are major contributors of vitamin C.

Vitamin D
Vitamin D is required to maintain normal development and function of bone, muscle, nerves and function of all cells of the body. Vitamin D helps to improve Polycystic Ovarian Syndrome (PCOS). Vitamin D helps to maintain fertility reserves in women. Vitamin D helps implantation of embryos. Vitamin D improves weak and low sperm count.

Where to find Vitamin D: The flesh of fatty fish (such as salmon, tuna, and mackerel) and fish liver oils are among the best sources. Small amounts of vitamin D are found in beef liver, cheese, and egg yolks. Some mushrooms provide vitamin D2 in variable amounts. Naturally, our skin converts sunlight to Vitamin D but less so in dark skin. People with dark skin should take additional vitamin D supplements.

Vitamin E.
Vitamin E is an anti-inflammatory vitamin. Vitamin E has been extensively studied, and it has become widely known as a powerful anti-oxidant that protects eggs and sperm from damage due to oxidants.

Where to find vitamin E: Vitamin E is available in a number of foods and plants, ranging from edible oils to nuts. Some vitamin E-containing foods include wheat, rice bran, barley, oat, coconut, palm and annatto. Other sources include rye, amaranth, walnut, hazelnut, poppy, safflower, maize and the seeds of grape and pumpkins. Vitamin E byproducts have also been detected in human milk and palm dates (Phoenix canariensis). Among the many sources of vitamin E are rice bran, palm oil and annatto oil.

Minerals and Proteins

Coenzyme Q10 (CoQ10)
CoQ10 slows down ageing and acts as an antioxidant. Coenzyme Q10, also known as CoQ10, is an antioxidant that is naturally found in the body. It can also be taken as a dietary supplement, and it has been recommended for some time as a supplement for men with low sperm count, low motility and other sperm-related problems.

Treatment with CoQ10 improves ovarian response to stimulation and treatment outcomes in young women with poor ovarian reserve.

Where to find CoQ10: Foods that provide CoQ10 are mainly animal products, dairy, poultry, and meat. Animal products like meat, fish, poultry, and milk are the best sources.

Gluthatione
First, let me expalin what oxidative stress is.

Oxidative stress is a bodily condition that happens when your antioxidant levels are low (See page on First Thing First for definitions). Anti-oxidant levels can be measured through your blood. When there is an imbalance of *oxidants* which is harmful, also known as *free radicals*, and *anti-oxidant, which is beneficial*, your body experiences *oxidative stress* (injury to cells and body organs). This imbalance can play a role in certain illnesses and conditions like diabetes and infertility.

Oxidative stress can lead to cell and tissue damage and breakdown. Oxidative stress has more harmful properties than helpful ones. It can break down cell tissue and cause DNA damage according to WebMD. Antioxidants play an important role in your body. They protect your body from free radicals, which become more widespread through oxidative stress. In turn, they can help protect cells from damage. This is where gluthatione comes in. Lack of *Glutathione* contributes to oxidative stress and plays a role in endometriosis and PCOS. Gluthathione protects the sperm from oxidative stress and damage.

Where to find glutathione: This powerful antioxidant is most plentiful in the red, pulpy area of the watermelon near the rind. It can also be found in broccoli, brussels sprouts, cabbage, cauliflower, spinach, and other cruciferous vegetables.

L-Carnitine (LC)

LC plays a crucial role in sperm production and maturation. They are related to sperm motility and have antioxidant properties. LC has the important function of regulating the oxidative state and status of the female reproductive system.

Where to find LC: Foods that provide carnitine are mainly animal products, dairy, poultry, and meat. Animal products like meat, fish, poultry, and milk are the best sources.

N-acetyl-cysteine (NAC)

NAC (a family of amino acid L-cysteine), is used mainly as an anti-oxidant (see glutathione above). NAC also contributes to glutathione manufacture and may help restore the dwindling pool of glutathione often caused by oxidative stress and inflammation. NAC use may improve sperm qualities and oxidative/antioxidant balance in infertile males.

NAC is an effective, cheap and safe to use in long standing unexplained infertility patients undergoing IUI. It improves pregnancy rate significantly. NAC is very useful in PCOS.

Where to find NAC: cruciferous vegetables, such as broccoli, cauliflower, brussels sprouts, and bok, choy allium vegetables, such as garlic and onions, eggs, legumes, lean protein, such as fish, and chicken.

DHEA

DHEA (also known as *dehydroepiandrosterone)* is a hormone produced by your body's adrenal glands. DHEA has been reported to improve pregnancy chances with diminished ovarian reserves.

Current best available evidence suggests that DHEA improves ovarian function, increases pregnancy chances and, by reducing aneuploidy (Note: Aneuploidy is the presence of an abnormal number of chromosomes in a cell) lowers miscarriage rates. DHEA over time also appears to improve fertility reserves in women. DHEA addition to fertility support is an effective option for patients with diminished ovarian reserves. DHEA supplements can be made from wild yam or soy.

Selenium

To really appreciate the importance of selenium, is to consider what its absence causes. Numerous reports connect selenium shortage in several reproductive and pregnancy-related problems. Low fertility and poor cell growth are associated with lack of selenium. In males, poor sperm count, low motility and abnormal sperm shapes are associated with low selenium content. Testosterone (the male hormone) production is affected by lack of selenium.

Where to find selenium: Seafood and organ meats are the richest food sources of selenium. Other sources include muscle meats, cereals and other grains, and dairy products

Omega-3 (also known as DHA.)

Omega-3 are essential for normal functioning and for the health of humans and all domestic animals. Omega-3 fatty acids found in some foods, have a wide-range of health benefits. The omega-3 intake results in higher antioxidant activity in human semen fluid and enhanced sperm count, sperm motility, and sperm shapes. Considerable number of infertile men with unknown cause of weak and low sperm count might benefit from omega-3 fatty acids administration.

Where to find Omega-3. Fatty fish. Fish and other seafood (especially cold-water fatty fish, such as salmon, mackerel, tuna, herring, and sardines). Nuts and seeds (such as flaxseed, chia seeds, and walnuts). Plant oils (such as flaxseed oil, soybean oil, and canola oil). Fortified foods (such as certain brands of eggs, yogurt, juices, milk, soy beverages, and infant formulas.

Essential Amino Acids.

Nine amino acids-histidine, isoleucine, leucine, lysine, methionine, phenylalanine, threonine, tryptophan, and valine-are not made by mammals and are therefore dietary essential or crucial nutrients. These are commonly called *essential amino acids*. They are essential for production, maturation and quality of both sperms and eggs.

Where to find Essential Amino Acids: Lysine is in meat, eggs, soy, black beans, quinoa, and pumpkin seeds.

Meat, fish, poultry, nuts, seeds, and whole grains contain large amounts of histidine.

Cottage cheese and wheat germ contain high quantities of threonine.

Methionine is in eggs, grains, nuts, and seeds.

Valine is in soy, cheese, peanuts, mushrooms, whole grains, and vegetables.

Isoleucine is plentiful in meat, fish, poultry, eggs, cheese, lentils, nuts, and seeds.

Dairy, soy, beans, and legumes are sources of leucine.

Phenylalanine is in dairy, meat, poultry, soy, fish, beans, and nuts.

Tryptophan is in most high-protein foods, including wheat germ, cottage cheese, chicken, and turkey.

Zinc
Zinc is necessary for the formation and ripening of sperms, for ovulation, and for fertilization. During pregnancy, lack of zinc causes a number of abnormities including abortion, premature baby, abnormal babies, and stunted growth.
Where to find zinc: Cashews, dry roasted, kidney beans, cooked, chicken breast roasted skin removed, almonds, dry roasted, peas, green, frozen, cooked, baked beans, canned, plain or vegetarian pumpkin seeds, dried, oysters and shell-fish.

Other key elements that play important roles in fertility and in particular in PCOS are *calcium and magnesium*. In addition, there is evidence that *metformin* (a medication to regulate blood sugar especially useful in PCOS), *resveratrol* (found in red grapes, useful in PCOS) and *melatonin* (a brain hormone important for control of sleep) act as anti-oxidants and anti-inflammatory agents. They are all fertility boosters. They all improve sperm quality in men and improve fertility in women with low ovarian reserves.

Chapter 9.
Herbs and Aphrodisiacs in Fertility and Reproductive Health

Warning: You should seek the support of a qualified herbalist or relevant medical practitioner before you use herbs. Use and misuse of herbs may result in serious clinical consequences.

Foods are herbs and some herbs are foods, the saying goes. Food and herbs can serve as medicines to treat illnesses and infertility. The next part of this book will inform you about fertility herbs and herbal aphrodisiacs that can enhance your fertility and sexual performance.

Fertility Herbs and Aphrodisiacs for Women and Men.
Vitex-Argnus Castus (also called Chasteberry)
This herb has antioxidant, anti-inflammatory and anti-infective actions amongst many others outside the reproductive system. Vitex can be used to treat some types of high prolactin disorder. High prolactin may stop ovulation, conception and implantation. Vitex also increases progesterone production, which is necessary to protect pregnancy from miscarriage. Vitex helps in relieving tensions and problems associated with menstrual periods.

Ashwagandha
Ashwagandha is an evergreen shrub that grows in Asia and Africa. The herb is used for stress. Ashwagandha supplements have been shown in some studies to benefit male fertility and increase testosterone levels. Ashwagandha treatment significantly increased sperm concentration, semen volume, and sperm motility in men with low sperm count. It

also increased sperm concentration and motility in men with normal sperm count. Ashwagandha improves sexual function in healthy women: improving orgasms, lubrication, satisfaction, and arousal. The herb reduces stress hormone cortisol and improve sleep.

Tribulus Terrestris {TT or Devil's Thorn. small calthrops (English), dagunro (Yoruba), and tisadu (Hausa)}
TT improves sexual urge in men and sperm production. It is also found to increase the levels of testosterone in men.

Ginkgo biloba ((In Yoruba: obi gbogbo nse).
Ginkgo extract, in women, may improve blood supply of uterus and ovaries after application to women with poor endometrial response during fertility treatment. It increases endometrial thickness. In men, injury to testes can be reversed by the herb. On the downside, it's considered that this herb may reduce sperm quality and its ability to penetrate an egg.

Lady's mantle
This herb is said to be beneficial by improving heavy period flow (menorrhagia) and prevention of early miscarriage.

Safed musli (Chlorophytum borivilianum, CB)
The roots of CB can be useful for the treatment of certain forms of sexual inadequacies, such as premature ejaculation and oligospermia in men.

Mondia whitei
It is used to increase sexual urge and for the management of low sperm count. Mondia improves total motility as well as progressive motility of sperm.

Date Palm (DPP, Phoenix dactylifera).
DPP seems to cure male infertility by improving the quality of sperm values such as sperm count, motility and shapes.

Maca (Lepidium meyenii)
An improvement in sexual desire has been observed with Maca. Maca oral administration significantly improves sexual performance in men. It is said that maca root helps women in menopause and also helps decrease premenstrual symptoms.

Moringa
This herb is said to be rich in vitamins B2 and B3, B6 and C, zinc, calcium, magnesium, phosphorus and folic acid. All of these are important for success in fertility especially also in PCOS.

Panax ginseng
The herb is said to have aphrodisiac activities by improving desire and sexual performance in men.

Black cohosh (BC)
Found in North America, BC is a member of the buttercup family. Benefits: it stimulates the release of LH and contains a substance called isoflavone that has estradiol effects (the female hormone).

Dong quai (DQ)
Native to China, it is used to strengthen weak uterus and regulate hormones and menstrual cycle. It may cause heavy bleeding during the menstrual periods.

Evening primose oil
This is found in Omega-3 and the benefit is to increase fertile cervical mucus. It should not be used after ovulation as it may cause uterine contractions.

False unicorn root
This is used for periods that have ceased (amenorrhoea) or thin, scanty periods (hypomenorrhoea), hormone imbalance and infertility issues.

Tonga Ali (Eurycoma longifolia)
Tonga Ali is used for erectile dysfunction (ED), male infertility, increasing sexual desire in healthy people, and boosting athletic performance, but there's no good scientific evidence to support most of these uses (WebMD).

Pausinystalia yohimbe
This an evergreen tree native to West Africa, also present in Asia. It is the only herb listed in the Physician's index reference for sexual function. Yohimbine is said to be a useful treatment option in erectile dysfunction.

Pycnogenol
Is an antioxidant plant extract that is found in the maritime pine in South West France. The extract is used to improve the functions of the sperm.

Wild Yam.
Wild yam is a good source for DHEA. Wild yam is also known to help with twinning and multiple pregnancies. It should be taken after ovulation as it may prevent ovulation if you take it before ovulation.

Red clover and *nettles* are said to be helpful to female fertility.

Chapter 10
Assisted Conception: Your Options Explained.

When you have tried all you can and conception success is not showing up naturally, then the time to seek outside help has come. Here is the medical *convention*: If you are a woman who is under 35years, you can try for a year before you ask for help. If you are over 35 years, ask for help after 6 months. Before you do any of these, try having penetrative vaginal sex 2 to 3 times per week. Or have sex during ovulation, 2 days before and 2 days after ovulation. The convention above is to guide us and help us manage infertility issues. In spite of the convention, individual circumstances differ. I have several clients and potential clients who would say: "I want to be pregnant fast…" "I want to get pregnant next month…" Or " …My husband is coming home from abroad and he has only 2 months to spend with me… I want to conceive while he is with me." The expressed desire may also go thus: "I got married 3 months ago, my husband is a sea fearer, I want to get pregnant immediately before he goes back to sea."

There was a case whereby a man (husband) was in prison. The man and his wife were agitating to have a child as the possibility of ever doing so was small with the husband serving a life sentence. The story went that the man's semen who was in prison, was collected and transported across international boundaries for the purpose of intra uterine insemination (IUI) of the wife. The procedure resulted in a pregnancy. In this case, desire, timing and personal circumstances made a ridicule of the convention. Obviously, in our setting and indeed in the world of infertility, if we ignore these pleas, the couple may simply go elsewhere where someone will listen and consider their desire. Therefore, in practical terms, the circumstances of each person and couple should be put into consideration individually and not, in modern times, be held down by archaic, impractical *convention*.

I once had a 26-year middle-class banker who came with her husband for fertility assistance. They had just recently married and were under pressure and with a message from grandparents, apparently, "to give me my grandchildren...I want to carry my grandchild." I applied the above convention and counselling. They left. Of course, they never came back. That is just one out of many cases.

In spite of trying naturally, if still there is no success, then it is time to see a fertility specialist. The specialist can be a Gynaecologist with interest in Fertility. A general gynecologist with no interest in fertility may not be helpful. Human Reproductionist is another specialist you should consider. The specialist may be a Reproductive Endocrinologist. It may also be an Andrologist: who deals with male's reproductive system. The specialist may be someone who combines all of the above. Your first point of call may be a nurse specialist, counsellor, psychologist or nutritionist who may provide counselling and further directions and referral to the appropriate physician. Similarly, your general medical practitioners (GP) will in most cases deal with some preliminary fertility issues such as advising you about change of life style, weight reduction and nutrition. If such suggestions are not working, then your GP should refer you to the appropriate specialist as mentioned above. Remember though, getting pregnant is one-step of the journey. Sustaining the pregnancy is another.

Seeing a specialist to achieve pregnancy is fertility intervention in one form or another. Fertility intervention can take many forms. In its simplest form, counselling or *therapy* without the use of medications may be all that an individual or a couple requires. *Counselling* has certainly worked for many of my clients. It takes the following forms. Reassuring the couple, avoiding relationship conflicts especially around ovulation may be all that is required. Also, taking a break, going out of your immediate home or state or environment to say, holiday resort or hotel at about the time of ovulation may help you conceive: provided you have lots of sex. This advice often results in a pregnancy. I also counsel couples to turn off their mobile phones and to concentrate on the "job" of intimacy and conception at hand. Focus is required.

A young couple in their late twenties came to see me around 2012. Childlessness was splitting their marriage. They could not see eye-to-eye even in my consultation room. They were backing each other when they came to see me. I then humbly asked them to sit and look at my eyes. They did. My "treatment" consisted only of counselling. "Go out with your wife sir. And ma, go out with your husband. Go to a hotel. Have good sex over the next 3 or 4 days." Having respected and accepted my advice, they left.

Two weeks after, the woman came back that she had missed her period. At first, I disbelieved her. In truth, she was pregnant. Counselling works.

Then, there is a couple who have had failed IUI in my clinic. Looking at their distress and financial squeeze, I said: "I am going to give you two months to go have good sex. Do it often. Target ovulation." As at the time of writing this book, the woman was 10 weeks pregnant: and already registered for antenatal care(ANC).

The advice or counselling can also take the form of education on *reverse Billing/Calendar* method of family planning.

In Billing's method of family planning, the couple and in particular the woman should know her ovulation or "unsafe" period when she can get pregnant. So, she avoids having sex during the unsafe periods. This is her time of ovulation. In *reverse Billings*, the couple should have sex, a lot of it, during and around the ovulation time.

Another form of fertility treatment is use of *medication*. This can come in form of taking simple supplements such as vitamins and minerals. These minerals supplements and vitamins may come in single packaging such as folic acid, iron, magnesium, vitamin D or C and so forth. They may come as a combination of several vitamins and minerals. They come in different brands. Several of our patients have benefited from this approach. My approach is to ensure all necessary fertility tests are done as a first step: to exclude possible underlying causes.

I once had a client whom I never set my eyes on but we communicated online. I instructed her to do the necessary tests. She did. No major findings. Then I suggested some branded supplements. Two months after our interaction, she sent me a message that she was pregnant.

Still, there was one, whose friend asked me to help. I never saw the client. On a sheet of paper, I wrote the vitamins and supplements she was to buy and use. A month or so after, I got a report from the same friend who introduced her, that she was pregnant.

In recent times, 2022 specifically, we have started to prescribe some brands that combine vitamins, amino acids and minerals. For several couples who has had lengthy problems with fertility, they got pregnant so quickly that I was almost in shock. Some of them were waiting on the line to have a more serious fertility treatment with very powerful drugs. In addition, almost all of them have had their full investigations done.

There are times that, *herbs will work* (see the chapter on herbs) and perhaps may be the only treatment that will work. In our practice, we combine herbs with vitamins and minerals to achieve results. I had a couple from USA whose case of poor sperm quality had caused him to be a write-off by his physician: Sperm motility was very poor. We gave herbs with minerals and vitamins for three months. Midway, we ordered for a repeat semen analysis: the quality had improved significantly. We also had given several clients herbs prior to other forms of assisted conception, to satisfactory outcomes.

Assisted conception can take different forms and shapes. We should not confuse Assisted Reproductive Technology (ART) with Assisted Conception. ART is nothing more than in-vitro fertilization (IVF). We will get into further details about IVF later in this chapter.

As I mentioned earlier, fertility treatment can take the form of prescription of more powerful fertility drugs to allow the ovaries to grow more eggs within a short period. Upon maturity, we then force multiple ovulations to occur over several days. In this method, many of our clients could get pregnant either during the procedure or subsequently within 2 to 3 months following. We call this procedure *superovulation.*

Intrauterine Insemination of Sperm or IUI for short (of either husband or donor's sperm) is a more direct form of assisting couples who wish to get pregnant. In this process, profession-ally prepared sperm of the husband or donor what we inject into the uterus of the woman at the time of ovulation. In our clinic, if the husband is the sperm donor and is able to, we encourage the couple to follow the IUI with more sex after-wards. Very often, IUI is for unexplained infertility (which occurs in about 10% of infertility population). IUI may be useful when the sperm quality is low. When sex is difficult or painful or when one couple is in a distant place, sperm can be collected and process for IUI.

ART and IVF.
IVF came into being with the birth of Louise Brown, on 25 July 1978. Thousands of individuals and couples around the world have benefited from IVF ever since. However, IVF is not for everyone. What works for X may not work for B. For one, IVF is causing highly unreasonable expectations. As a result, we have seen candidates seeking fertility treatment asking online and in office, in a tone that tends to portray IVF as a retail or off-the-shelf item that you can buy at will: "I want to do IVF…How much are you doing your IVF?" Some will say: "How much is your IVF?" After counselling and af-ter comprehensive investigations, they frequently conceive naturally or get pregnant with lesser fertility treatment than IVF would have offered. Some will intentionally delay con-ception with the belief that: "I am not ready to get pregnant now. If I can't conceive when I am ready, I will simply do IVF." Fertility treatment should be according what the person needs and each person should receive the appropriate solution that will address the problem. My approach is while IVF is reassuring; it is not the solution for all infertility issues.
In fact, I believe that a fertility treatment should start with the simplest form that meets the individual person's needs. No need to go straight from the start to IVF.

IVF is very expensive all over the world. However, IVF and its many sister variants such as intracytoplasmic sperm injection (ICSI) may be the last resort if all other forms of fertility treatments have failed. It may also be that IVF is the only viable option considering your circumstances.

I have had the opportunity to see and happily too, couples whose IVFs failed but who subsequently conceived naturally on their own. We can say the same thing for IUI too.

Gender Selection (Family Balancing): As the law of each country may allow for gender selection, this can be achieved through IVF and IUI. There are some natural though unproven methods to achieve a male or female baby to "balance" the family.

Genetic Screening and Selection: Many genetic illnesses put would-be parents and fertility physicians under pressure and in dilemma. Example is sickle cell disease (SCD). If a couple consists of each one carrying the AS gene, there is a high chance that their child or children conceived naturally, could end up as AS or SS or AA genotypes.

To avoid the scenario of having an SS child, the choices of a fertility treatment may be AA-gene carrier sperm donor or egg donor of AA genes. This may be unacceptable to the couple who wish to have "our own biological children". Solutions and technology to address this issue is at the moment limited. Therefore, pre-pregnancy screening or pre-pregnancy diagnosis or testing means the couple will first have an IVF. Following this, each of their embryos will undergo screening to see if any of the embryo carries SS gene. All SS embryos are removed and non-SS are transferred to the couple or their surrogate.

71

This procedure is expensive and risky. Couples should consider their options carefully. Further, the best approach is to avoid this scenario in the first instance by screening your partner carefully before commitment in a relationship or childbearing.

Fertility Rejuvenation (Fertility Boosting)
For women who have had early menopause (complete stoppage of periods before age of 45 years or premature ovarian dysfunction which is on and off stoppage of your period before the age of 45 years, it is now possible to reverse this condition is some cases. Still, in some women whose fertility reserves have fallen below that which we expect of their age, fertility rejuvenation procedure may help. The goal is to improve egg yield, to "wake up" a failing ovary for the purpose of conception, or to delay the onset of menopause. We have had, in our practice, some successes in these regards.
This process is similarly applicable to men who suffer from low sperm count.

Egg freezing has taken off in recent times. If you intend to delay conception or you are undergoing chemotherapy or radiation for cancer or some other reasons, you may consider egg freezing. *Sperm and embryo freezing* are already part of fertility services in most fertility centres.

Chapter 11
New Developments and the Future.

The future of fertility treatment is wide open and new researches are bringing in new opportunities to address some troubling issues I will address below.

Crispr (Clustered Regularly Interspaced Short Palindromic Repeats) or Gene Editing.
This is a form of technology that helps us to remove abnormal genes that may cause disease.

Gene editing has been used in an experimental way to prevent HIV from infecting a baby. Other trials have successfully used CRISPR to knock out troubling genes. That technique has improved the symptoms of sickle cell disease in at least three sufferers. So, there is hope in the future for dealing with genetic diseases such as sickle cell disease.
The application in future, may hopefully help infertile persons who inherited some abnormal genes from their family (see Chapter One). An example is premature ovarian failure and dysfunction in women or azoospermia and oligospermia in men.

Postpone your menopause is a form of new treatment whereby you can freeze a part of your ovaries while you are young and healthy. Then, later, such frozen tissue is returned to the ovary to start growing and producing hormones. With this, you delay your menopause and extend your fertility potentials. There are recent reports of babies being conceived and delivered using this form of treatment.

Uterus (Womb) transplant is now a reality. I used to dream of this type of treatment as a young doctor during my training years. Now, women without uterus can have one. Some have had conception and delivery following womb transplant.

Section 4
Frequently Asked Questions

"The key to wisdom is this – constant and frequent question-
ing, for by doubting we are led to question, by questioning
we arrive at the truth."
– Peter Abelard

Chapter 12
Most Frequently Asked Questions and Comments In Fertility, Gyanecology and Andrology. Part One.

The following questions, comments and inquiries are real and from individuals and couples who have had trouble with fertility or gynaecology and andrology. We received them and printed them here with some minor modifications. They are frequently recurring issues that appear to be at the top of the minds of the persons concerned. Embarrassingly, these are not issues or questions that patients even within the confidentiality and privacy of a physician in a consulting room may offer willingly. We are grateful that we have access to these questions. We appreciate the trust these individuals have in us. That said, some of these questions have been dealt with elsewhere in the book.

1. ***"How can I boost my fertility?"***
   This is from a woman. The answer to this question depends on the current level of fertility reserve in the case of each person. Generally, if the reserve is low, some of the drugs and supplements discussed in the book under "Vitamins and Supplements" will help. Examples: Omega-3, DHEA in combination with others will improve low reserve.
   An additional step is to consider ovarian rejuvenation. Exercises, good nutrition and good sleep are essential to boosting fertility alongside removal of infections. For men, we have successfully used some of the vitamins, supplements and herbs in various combinations to boost male fertility while infection is also treated and we treat any underlying illness.

2. ***"What steps should I take to boost my fertility? I am TTC."*** *(*Answer applicable to women and men).
1. Avoid all infections in your reproductive pathway. Urgently treat all existing infections in your reproductive tract.

2. Keep your BMI (Body-Mass-Index) within range 18-25.

3. Exercise 150 mins per week (aerobics, anaerobics, and stretching and resistance exercises).

4. Eat simple balanced natural diets and take adequate amount (3 to3.5L) of good water daily.

5. Avoid toxins: alcohol, nicotine/cigarettes, plastics, other pollutants/toxins in air, food, water, cosmetics and pharmaceuticals. Go natural.
.
6. Treat all existing illnesses such as infections, blocked tubes, fibroid, endometriosis, diabetes, thyroid disorders and other hormones imbalances.

7. Avoid stress, whatever it takes and have good sleep.

8. Monitor your ovulation and have a lot of sex at your ovulation window.

9. Routinely take folic acid and multivitamins much before and during pregnancy.
.
10. Act to have children within natural time range. Nothing lasts forever. Make hay while the sun shines.

Time is everything. If not possible for any reason to conceive, seek medical help early. Do not delay.

3. *"What herbs can I use to boost my fertility?"*
For women, individual circumstances differ. There are various combinations of herbs or even individual hers such as Vitex in women and Ashwagandha that may improve fertility in women and men. Some branded ones are also available. See the Chapter on herbs for more.

4. *"All my tests are normal. But I am not getting pregnant. Why?"*
It is frustrating knowing that all of your tests are normal, yet you are not getting pregnant. This condition in called "unexplained infertility." You are not alone. 15% to 30% of couples who desire a child fall into the group of unexplained infertility. However, half of such couples who suffer from fertility of unknown cause will conceive within one year of trying to get pregnant. I have to say that there is no smoke without fire.
Taking fertility boosters: minerals with vitamins and changing lifestyle, nutrition, sleep, more targeted sex, less friction in the relationship, losing weight and exercising may help you to get pregnant.

5. *"How can I boost my eggs?"*
You can boost your eggs as earlier stated.

6. *"How can I boost my sperms?"*
   You can boost your sperms if you exercise regularly, treat all infections, take the vitamins and supplements that we recommend, avoid heating up your testes via the use of laptops or hot water bath, tight trousers and leg crossing. Avoid watching TV beyond 10 pm; avoid placing mobile phone close to your testes. Eat nuts and balanced meals. Lose weight. Avoid harmful drugs, alcohol, and cigarette/nicotine and treat any underlying illnesses.

7. *"I have fathered 2 children. I am fertile. Do I need any fertility test?"*
   This is a wrong assumption. On the face of it, we age every day. Our bodies are affected by toxins, infections and by our behavior. What was true a month ago with regards to our fertility may no longer be true today. Our fertility quality changes as we age.

8. *"When should I meet my husband for conception during my cycle?"*
   To achieve conception, couples should be involved sexually at least 2 to 3 times per week. This is random sex. For more focused and targeted meeting, sex should occur 2 days before ovulation, during ovulation and 2 days after ovulation. This calls for you to know your fertile period or ovulation time.

9. *"What causes sperm flow back after sex"?*
   This has been explained in the book.

10. *"I don't have orgasm during sex. Am I normal?"*
    According to Royal College of Obstetricians and Gynaecologists, 54 % of women have trouble with sex

at some point. Some estimation put it that 80% of women do not experience orgasm. This does not mean that you are abnormal. The issue is inadequate sexual stimulation. With sufficient stimulation, orgasm can occur. In as much as orgasm helps move sperm forward towards uterus, orgasm is not a necessary condition for achieving conception. Note though, female circumcision may seriously decrease the chance of reaching orgasm in such a woman.

11. *"I am blood O negative. My husband is A positive. I had a miscarriage 2 years ago but I didn't get anti-D. Is this why I am finding it difficult to conceive again?"*

Broadly, human blood groups can be divided into two classes; Positive and Negative. Strange as it may seem to us, this sorting is based on a specific finding in our blood that we share with Rhesus Monkeys.

If a person has positive blood group, that person has marker in his or her blood cell surface that he or she shares with the monkey: and that individual is Rhesus Positive. Otherwise, such person is Negative.

A mother who is negative, may without fear carry a negative baby from a negative father without much risk.

A mother who is negative may carry a positive baby but with a real risk of blood reactions in the mother. Such reactions may affect the baby in the womb in subsequent pregnancies but not in a current pregnancy. A negative mother should not get a positive blood transfusion.

Tests:
Your medical doctor preferably, a gynaecologist, will decide along with a haematologist, the range of tests to do to weigh your risks against your next pregnancy.

Prevention:
Immunoglobulin injection (Anti-D) at 28 and 34 weeks or just at 28-week pregnancy only may prevent reactions. If there is suspicion of reaction having occurred, a preventive injection called immunoglobulin should be given within 72 hours at the birth of the child or miscarriage or blood transfusion. Nothing can be done outside this time to neutralize a formed antibody reaction.

Effect on conception: Not having or never been given Anti-D does not impair conception but may affect survival of the baby.
If you have missed Anti-D, go straight now to your gynaecologist or general practitioner.

12. *"Which sex position is best for conception?"*
The whole idea of having sex is primarily to enable sperm from the male to meet the egg from the female. If the conditions are right, the following positions will enhance the chances of conception:
● Male on top (missionary) with aim of depositing the semen close to the cervix.

●Back access into vagina.

●The recipient (female) raises her legs or places them on the walls. This last point allow push up of sperm into the uterus.

13. "I do not see stretchy cervical mucus during ovulation or do I not ovulate? How can I improve my cervical mucus to be friendly to sperm?"

The big question is: Can you ovulate without seeing the vaginal discharge due to cervical mucus?

Much discussion has been made of cervical mucus discharge as a mark of ovulation. Many individuals rely on this to confirm or be reassured of ovulation.

Note that:

1. What works for X may not work for W.

2. A mark or sign of ovulation in one person may not necessarily appear in everyone.

3. The validation of ovulation may require you to combine temperature change with, slight pelvic pain with cervical mucus discharge plus breast tenderness at the time of ovulation even with a little mood change.

Recall, individuals are different.

In sum, the absence of one symptom is not to say ovulation has not occurred.

Healthy cervical mucus is crucial to natural conception. Increase your chances by consuming foods rich in vitamin B and by drinking a lot of water. You should treat and avoid all forms of infections. Stress yourself less. Sleep well.

14. *"What is causing my heavy period?"*

Your heavy period is due to something like:
- Fibroid
- Hormone imbalance
- PCOS
- Drugs and herbs
- Thyroid and blood disorders

15. *"Why is my period so painful?"*

A painful period may be innocent and as part of growing up and maturing. We call this type primary dysmenorrhoea. This is often associated with women who are yet to get pregnant and deliver except that endometriosis may also be a cause

However, when it is not primary, it's secondary and this type is often due to infections or pelvic inflammatory disease (PID), endometriosis, adenomyosis (period flow into the body of the womb) and some types of ovarian cysts such as dermoid cysts (dermoid cyst is a type of cyst in the ovary).

16. *"What is causing my period to be thin, dark and like a drop? It sometimes last less than 2 days?"*

Your scanty periods could be due to any of the following?
- Thin endometrium
- Uterine adhesions (womb lining getting stuck together)
- Low blood levels (anaemia)
- Drugs and hormone use
- Hormone imbalance.

There are various solutions and procedures that your specialist doctor can advise including the use of herbs to improve endometrial thickness. Solutions have been mentioned earlier.

17. *"What causes PCOS?"*

PCOS stands for polycystic ovarian syndrome: is a wide and complicated issue. PCOS affects many women about 10-15% of women and one in every four of infertility population. Some women are not even aware that they are victims of this very common and complex disorder.
.
What causes PCOS?

●Inheritance. About 3.5% of PCOS can pass on from family members. This is an inherited form of PCOS.
●Hormone disruptors: Environmental toxins and pollution such as air pollution, petrochemicals and plastics and some home cooking items.
●Pesticides
●Some cosmetics and beauty products.
●Autoimmune disorders
●There is associations of thyroid disorders and PCOS
●Other organs may be involved such as adrenal gland.

Some effects of PCOS:
●Irregular periods /hormone imbalance
●Infertility
●Diabetes may occur
●Weight gain
●Unwanted body hairs, greasy skin and acne
●Depression, anxiety, anger, unstable mood.
●Sexual difficulties and vaginal dryness

Some ideas on managing PCOS: Regular exercises including resistance exercises, taking the vitamins and supplements suggested earlier. Change in your food content is key to helping with PCOS.

18. *"Can you help me remove my womb adhesion so I can conceive?"*

Womb adhesions or sometimes called by name of the person who first described the condition: Asherman's, is the womb equivalent of blocked fallopian tubes. Nothing may pass through blocked or adhered uterine walls linings. Womb adhesion may be a result of infection (tuberculosis) and operation to remove an unwanted pregnancy. It may result from previous surgery in the womb such as fibroid operation or other procedures.

Conception, sperm movements and menstrual periods may not happen because of uterine adhesions.

There are solutions available to deal with this issue.

19. *"Why am I not ovulating?"*

For conception to occur, (follicular or) egg development is not enough. You must ovulate whatever it takes and the egg must get fertilized. The resulting embryo should be transported into the womb where growth continues. We explained all of these in earlier chapters of this book.

Causes of failure to ovulate are:

1a. Extremes of ages of reproduction: few years after onset on your periods, ovulation may be erratic as the hormones settle down and later stabilize. At menopause which is a permanent cessation of your periods and few years before menopause, ovulation becomes erratic.

1b. Premature ovarian failure or dysfunction (this is when an ovary that fails before you reach age of 45) which may occur at any age.

2. Hormone imbalance issues such as high prolactin
3. Ovarian disorders such as PCOS especially.

4. Menstrual disorders such as endometriosis may affect ovulation.
5. Absence of ovaries from birth.
6. Absence or reduced function of ovaries due to surgery.
7. Medications and family planning hormones may suppress ovulation.
8. Treatments or exposure to chemotherapy or radiotherapy may impair the ovaries.
9. Stress, depression or mental health issues and their medications may suppress ovulation.
10. Other illnesses affecting the brain, thyroid, adrenals, kidney and liver may impair the function of your reproductive hormones.
11. Infection like mumps in childhood or at other times and adult infection affecting the ovaries. Other problems like pelvic inflammatory disease (PID) may cost you ovulation.
12. Genetic/Chromosomal Disorders such as Turners Syndrome.
If you are not ovulating, something has gone wrong in the normal course of events and you should see your medical specialists for assistance.

20. *"Why am I so dry during sex? Can you help me?"*

Lovemaking (sex) is an essential part of human re-production. It is a crucial stage in the process of conception and pleasure and bonding of partners.

However, for enjoyable sex to occur, vaginal wetness should occur. Failing, sex may become difficult and painful for the partners.

What causes dryness?

- Hormonal imbalance
- Fear, depression and anxiety
- Pelvic surgery especially removal of ovaries.
- Medications
- Aging and Menopause
- Poor foreplay / inadequate stimulation.

Poor vaginal lubrication may affect sperm movement and reduce chances of conception. If the dryness is not due to any medical issue above, water-based lubricants that are friendly to the sperm may help.

21. *"Why can't I reach orgasm during sex?"*

Lack of orgasm (Anorgasmia) can be primary (never had orgasm) or secondary (had orgasm before but no more) or based on situation. Common causes of orgasm problems in women include:

- Failure to get enough stimulation (foreplay).
- Fear of failure in sexual performance
- Mental health disorders, such as depression and anxiety
- Physical Illnesses: Examples chronic pain condition such as arthritis
- Atrophy of clitoris (natural, chemical or surgery or due to disuse, hormonal changes, and lack of blood flow to the clitoris).

●History of traumatic sexual experience such as abuse and rape.

●Difficulties and unresolved conflicts in relationship.

●Problems with hormones: Low sex hormones like estradiol and testosterone.

●Medications: Examples are antidepressants in the class of selective serotonin reuptake inhibitors (SSRIs).

●Alcohol

●Pelvic surgery: Gynaecological surgery. Example is hysterectomy or vaginal surgery.

●Medical conditions: Examples are heart disease that limit sexual performance and diabetes that may have damaged nerves.

●Cultural or religious beliefs that sex is not good or causing guilt feelings

●Shyness

●Poor body image

●Guilt about enjoying sexual activity

●Substance misuse: alcohol and smoking

●Female circumcision of clitoris and other genital parts mutilation.

●Situational Anorgasmia:

The commonest type of orgasm problem occurs when you can only come to orgasm during particular settings such as during masturbation.

Solutions: The solution will depend on what is causing the lack of orgasm. Such solution may include training, psychological treatment, surgical procedures, rejuvenation and medications as the case may be. You can conceive without having orgasm.

"My husband is AS and I am AS, what can we do to avoid having SS child?"

Sickle cell disease is the commonest genetic disorder in people of African descent.

In Nigeria, 2.2% of the population suffers from the SS disorder, which brings huge pain and distresses to the victim and the family. The problems include, pain, crisis, low blood amongst others.

Still 25% of the population are carriers or AS and do not in general, suffer crisis except under certain conditions.

How can you avoid having a sickle cell child (SCD)?

Note: Mathematically, AS+AS parents have 1:4 chances of a SCD child. But if there are 4 kids, all 4 children can be AS, AA or SS in reality. Same permutation applies to SC+AS.

In another combination: AC + AS partners: You stand to have AA, SC, AC and AS mathematically. In a 4-children set, all may be AA or SC or AC or AS or mixed.

What can you do?

1. From the start, make a good choice of partners. Do not take the risk. The maths may not favour you.

2. Thoroughly check the genotype and or genetic makeup of your partners in at least THREE

CREDIBLE laboratories before you marry or have a child at all. Then make your informed choice.

3. If you are already married, then the following are your choices:

4a) If pregnant: Do chorionic villus sampling (CVS) at 1st to 2nd (up to 20 weeks) trimester of pregnancy. There are side effects. You may decide to terminate the pregnancy if the child is SCD.

b). You can do Amniocentesis in the second tri-mester. Sample of amniotic fluid is taken for analysis. There are side effects too and termination of pregnancy is an option.

A new test in which all that is required is the blood sample from the mother is being developed. Not ready for wider use yet.

5. Before you get pregnant: Engage IVF or fertility doctors to screen the embryo and select embryo that are not carrying SS gene for transfer.

6. New technology now exists to select sperms that are identified as not carrying S gene for purposes of fertilisation during IVF. This process may not be so useful for IUI.

None of these choices come easily. But think of cost of having a SCD child.

22. *"Why is my womb lining thin?"*
Your womb lining (endometrium) could be thin if your eggs are not producing enough of the female hormone called estradiol. It's estradiol that thickens the womb lining (endometrium). Your womb lining could be thin if the womb itself is not responding as it should to the call of estradiol. If you have had surgery or "D & C" procedure in the past, it may have resulted in damaging the womb lining and restricting its ability to renew and grow new lining. Drugs and herbs and hormone family planning methods may thin out the womb linings. Low blood level of any kind, may cause thin womb linings.

23. *"Can you open my blocked tubes without surgery?"*

Every individual circumstance differs. Some tubal blockages may open up upon non-surgical intervention. Some others will require surgery. In our practice, we have been able to open up blocked tubes without surgery and some got pregnant following the procedure.

24. *"Can I be pregnant and still be having my periods?"*
The short and long answer to this question is that these two conditions of pregnancy and regular periods are unlikely to occur together.

That said, the following possibilities are likely causes of bleeding in pregnancy that may be confused with periods:

In the first 2-3 weeks of pregnancy, a condition called implantation bleeding may occur. This bleeding is small and nothing comparable to normal period. It stops on its own. But for women with scant and short periods, this may be confusing. A valid pregnancy test will help sort the issue out.

Bleeding from say 4-5 weeks onward is more likely to be threatening miscarriage.

Other likely causes of bleeding you may confuse with "period" are:

●Cancer of cervix, vagina, vulva that exist together with pregnancy.

●Polyps (innocent growth) of cervix

●Bleeding disorders not related to pregnancy.

●Sexual trauma.

●In the rare case of double uterus where pregnancy is in one.

From second trimester onward, the following may occur.

●Low-lying placenta that bleeds from time to time may be confused with occurrence of periods. *Solutions:*

Get pregnancy test done and get a comprehensive assessment by a Gynaecologist.

Bleeding is a serious issue at any time and a threat to life. Do not delay in seeking help.

25. *"How do I get pregnant?* Another version of the question is *"How can I get pregnant fast?"*

This question may seem simplistic and even amusing. However, it is not funny to the person asking. Even natural sexual encounter is a stranger to some.

The most obvious answer is that sperm (male) must meet the egg (female) no matter what it takes and by whatever means. That is the surest way to obtaining conception.

Thus, available methods to getting pregnant are:

•Natural sexual encounter with your partner. The female egg must meet the male sperm before you can conceive.

Some help from fertility doctors may help you. Examples:

•Superovulation

•IUI

•IVF

•Counselling with or without medications

•You may require a surgery to remove barriers before you could get pregnant.

26. *"Can I ovulate twice in the same cycle?"*

Is it possible to ovulate at multiple times at different occasions or more than once in same menstrual cycle month?

A research report in Fertility and Sterility Journal in 2003 addressed this question. Also, a lot of questions and comments about "stretching mucus" at different times in the same cycle by our inquiring clients seem to confirm the possibility of multiple ovulations in the same cycle.

This is not surprising: we have many non-identical twins in Nigeria and we consume a lot of cassava and yams, all of which, its believed, may contribute to hyper ovulation or multiple ovulation. Your genetic makeup is another factor that may cause multiple ovulation (hyper ovulation). Multiple ovulations can happen in PCOS persons or individuals who recently stopped using oral contraceptive pill type of family planning. Hyper ovulation is different from superovulation.

What of Superovulation?

This is multiple ovulations that occur at about the same time or close to each other. This is usually due to fertility treatments or drugs to bring about many ovulations.

The risk of hyper ovulation is not being able to predict ovulation or pregnancy. Multiple pregnancies can also occur at different times of the month.

For superovulation: multiple pregnancies are huge possibilities and excessive egg growth also called ovarian hyper stimulation syndrome may occur during fertility treatment.

27. *"When is the best time to start antenatal care (ANC) when you are pregnant?"*
This is a common question that lingers in the mind of expectant mothers as we do get this inquiry so frequently.

There is no fixed time. The rule of thumb is to start as soon as your pregnancy is confirmed by an ultrasound or if your pregnancy test is positive.

Starting early has huge benefits such as:

Your pregnancy can be confirmed early including where the pregnancy is located (to exclude ectopic pregnancy). You can also determine the number of foetuses.

The age of the pregnancy is best determined in the first 13 weeks of pregnancy.

The expected delivery date (EDD) can be calculated if you start early.

Existing illnesses or diseases can be tackled early before they take root and affect your baby and yourself. Potential illnesses such as anaemia (low blood levels) can be prevented early. Relationship can be established with a care team to aid with proper care.

Imagine the following scenario; All of the following affected individuals should as a matter of priority register early, as soon as possible.

● This is your first pregnancy regardless of your age.
● You are older than 35 and this is your first pregnancy.
● You have had more than 4 children.
● You had previous assistance or operation to deliver a child.
● You had assisted conception leading to this pregnancy.
● You had previous traumatic delivery such as premature delivery, lots of bleeding before or after delivery etc.

- You have had multiple pregnancy losses.
- You had a pelvic operation lately.
- You have existing medical disorders such as high blood pressure now, before or during last pregnancy, diabetes and other medical issues.

28. *"How many times can I use post-pill (Emergency Contraception) in a cycle month?"*

Similar question: ***"I used post-pill this cycle but I am not seeing my period. I did PT but its negative?"***

The artificial hormone called levonorgestrel is a form of female hormone called progesterone which is contained in both brands called "Postinor 1" which has one tablet or "Postinor 2" that has two tablets.

This version of levonorgestrel (artificial progesterone) is used as an emergency family planning. Either Postinor 1 or Postinor 2 must be used within 72 hours of unprotected sex.

In Postinor 2, the second tablet should be used 12 hours after the first tablet.

How often should Postinor (a brand) or this type of emergency contraceptive be used in a cycle?

Generally, once is recommended.

Side effects: The major side effect especially if you use this medication more than once in a cycle is the disruption of the menstrual cycle. The cycle can become irregular and ovulation become unpredictable.

Benefits: This type of emergency family planning is highly effective but not advisable for regular use.

Instead, consider a more stable and effective contraception if you are not yet ready for pregnancy.

29. *"I am a 29-year old virgin. I am getting married in 2 months. Should I be worried about sex? What do I need to know?"*

Enough to say, that virginity or celibacy is not a sin.

Medically, it is a fact that early sex in life (teens) leads to early sexually transmitted infection, PID, blocked tubes and hence infertility. Careless sex has medical consequences such as unwanted pregnancies and guilt: all of these are avoided when you keep your virginity.

Introduction to Sex: What You Should Know:

Cooperation of the two partners are absolutely necessary. This will push the fertility and sex hormones into action.

Total privacy is necessary. No distraction at all. Noise/music or sex in darkness or light is a choice to that you can agree in a romantic way with your partner.

A good body odour (or smell) is desirable.
A decent and clean environment is essential.

Foreplay and caressing and no rushing (especially by the man) of each other is essential.

It is important that the female be in control of sex so you can have satisfaction. Control the speed.

Vaginal lubrication is important. Due to sex hormones, lubrication is the secretion of fluid into the vagina during sex. Without adequate lubrication, sex may be difficult.

Upon invitation by female, the man should go gently by introducing the penis into the vagina. To gain entry for the first time, several gentle attempts at vaginal entry may be required. No force to enter, no rushing so as to avoid injuries, frustration and pain.

Success at vaginal entry may not come at first trial. Try another time and another time. One step at a time. Success may be another day. Try again. But the man should not be in hurry. The woman should open her legs as wide as possible to allow the penis to enter the vagina.

On vaginal entry, gentle penile thrusting is required.

Climaxing (also known as "come", orgasm) leads to release of semen by male. The female has intense sense of heightened pleasure. Be aware you may get pregnant even at the first time of having sex.
Partners are satisfied. Partners should remain together in bed and not rush to the exit door.
After a while, clean up or go for more rounds. Enjoy your life.

30. *"Why do I have a bad vaginal odour? My husband is complaining. What can I do Dr?"*

First Things First:

The vagina by nature is a fluid producing organ located in a space that prevents open ventilation. At the same time, the job that the vagina does allows it to be moist and humid. This is a perfect environment for bacteria to flourish. Normally, these bacteria are protective.

There are occasions when unfriendly bacteria may live in the vagina and therefore cause problems.

Causes of vaginal bad odour:
With this in mind, bad odour may develop even in normal circumstances such as:
Heat, humid and sweating time.
After sex (remember: sperm smells too).
Hormonal changes during menstrual cycle.

Abnormal conditions that cause vaginal odour:
Bacterial vaginosis — excessive growth of normal bacteria in vaginal area— is a common cause of vaginal odour.
Sexually transmitted infection(STI/STD): Trichomoniasis may cause vaginal odour.
Note: other STDs like yeast or gonorrhoea may not cause vaginal odour.
Inflammation of vagina: vaginitis may cause odour.
Poor personal hygiene could cause offensive odour.
Cancer of the cervix and the vagina.
Leakage of urine from the bladder or fistula between the bladder and the vagina.
Leakage of faeces (poo) between the rectum and the vagina.
Sanitary pads or tampons left in the vagina.
Prevention:
Personal hygiene is of utmost importance.

Allowing ventilation in the pelvic area.
Avoid douching and steaming.

31. ***"I am pregnant. When can I check the gender (sex) of my baby?"***
Traditionally, you wait until birth before you know the sex or gender of your baby. Even at this, some ambiguities still exist.

Next, you can wait until 18-20 weeks for mid-trimester ultrasound to determine the sex. In general, the ultrasound for gender can be from 14 weeks.

About accuracy of ultrasound gender determination:

A study by Manette Kearin and colleagues in Australas J Ultrasound Med revealed:

"Results confirmed 100% accuracy in predictions made after a 14 week gestation period. The overall success rate in the first trimester group (11–14 weeks) was 75%. When excluding those scans where a prediction could not be made, success rates increased to 91%. Results were less accurate for foetuses younger than 12 weeks, with an overall success rate of 54%."

In our practice, we normally wait for 20 weeks for gender determination by ultrasound.

A new blood test can now be used to confirm gender from the 7th week of pregnancy. Accuracy 98%. This is very expensive.

Some urine tests: Not very accurate: About 40% accuracy.

"In comparison, tests that analyzed DNA from urine instead of blood were only accurate 41 percent of the time" (LiveScience).

Summary:
Do IVF and PGT to determine gender before you get pregnant at all. This is not cheap.

Try the expensive blood test from the 7th week. Combine above or wait until 18-20 weeks for an ultrasound.

32. *"Why am I itching so much? I have treated thrush but the itching is not going away. Help me Dr. Vulva and indeed vagina itching is a common complaint."*

Causes of vulva (or vulvo-vagina) itching

Vulva Itching;
●Sexually transmitted infection (STI) such as Chlamydia, genital herpes, genital warts, trichomoniasis, gonorrhea and other organisms may cause vaginal/vulva itching as well as irritation. Other symptoms may also develop.

●Commonly, an infection such as candidiasis (also called yeast or thrush) is responsible in most cases either during pregnancy or not.

●Bacteria Vaginoses

●Some parasites could lead to itching: scabies and worms especially in circumstances where personal hygiene is poor or in crowded places such as school dorms for your girls.

●Lichen sclerosis which is seen in middle age women

●Cancer of vulva

●Drug allergy such as chloroquine etc.

●Tampons, pads condoms etc. may cause vaginal or vulva itching too

●Anxiety, depression or other mental health disorders may cause fixation on vulvo-vagina area as well as accompanying itching.

●Hormonal changes with low estrogen seen in later reproductive end. Breast feeding may cause low estrogen too or family planning preparations.

Stubborn or recurring itching: causes---

Itching that refused to go away should be well evaluated in view of the likely causes such as:

●Diabetes mellitus

●Poor or wrong treatment of the itching in first instance.

●Drug resistance

●Reinfection from sexual contacts.

Solution:
Try and identify the cause and avoid it.

A visit to the gynaecologist for treatment should be in order.

Preventions:
Keep vagina and vulva area well ventilated.
Keep personal hygiene perfect.
Be aware of and avoid sexually transmitted infections.

33. *"When should I meet my husband during my cycle for conception? I am TTC"*

There is a lot of evidence that unplanned sexual encounters result in pregnancies. This random system seems to be the way nature wants it to be for several reasons: including couple bonding, pleasure of sex and not being under pressure to conceive.

Time & Timing: "For purposes of conception"

For couples that are struggling with sex, time, distance, delay in conception and being under pressure to conceive, a more focused, and timed sexual encounter may be the way.

In that case: sex around ovulation may be appropriate. Start 2 -3 days before / through ovulation and continue 1-2 days after ovulation. Sperm life span is 3-5 days in the human body once discharged. The egg is only 24 hours. The more quality sperm around the egg, the greater chance of success. The first 12 to 18 hours of an egg's life is crucial and ideal for conception.

For individuals with irregular periods, kindly follow our advice on tracking your ovulation article. In brief, take your temperature daily: a rise of 0.2 to 0.5C indicates ovulation in absence of illness. Combine this temperature rise with mild pelvic pain, tingling breast, mood changes, slight vaginal blood spotting or the classic stretching cervical mucus discharge.

To be successful, sperm or semen must be good. Ovaries, fallopian tubes and the womb must work without problems. Merely having sex is not enough. Timing is not sufficient too if other barriers exist on the way.

34.

"If I masturbate, does that change my virginity? Can I have a repair to my hymen?"
The answers to these questions are matters of law, custom, science and medicine. Need we add religion?

So, we are going to tow a very thin line passing through a massive unnecessary controversy.

In sum, a virgin is someone, in the case of a woman, who has not had a pubic or vaginal encounter with a penis. A penis that touches the most peripheral part of the pubis makes the female and male partners non-virgin: this is regardless of the presence or absence of the hymen.

Hymen is that thin membrane from birth, which may cover the outer edges of the vagina.
Hymen may naturally be present and cover the vagina entry point completely or partially as leftovers.
It's a most unreliable signal to prove virginity especially if it's already torn naturally or through non-

sexual meddling such as masturbation, surgery or introduction of a foreign object.

A complete hymen can only prove that no object, penis or otherwise have passed through the complete and untorn hymen. A torn hymen proves nothing.
As we can now see, hymen is not helpful in proving virginity.

Can a torn hymen be repaired or be repairable? It is highly unlikely. It is even almost impossible.
Can masturbation change virginity? From the above-mentioned, it seems highly unlikely that self- masturbation has impact on virginity.

35. *"Is staphylococcus aureus (s.aureus) a sexually transmitted infection? How can I get rid of it? Can it affect my fertility? I need help."*
To keep it simple, s. aureus is a class of bacteria that is extremely widely distributed.
They are part of human normal bacteria found in our nostrils, breathing spaces and our skin.
Normally, the bacteria does not cause us problems.

However, they do as opportunists by taking advantage of our weak points.
Hence, they can cause, chest infection and boils on our skin as well as cause eye, nose, urine infections to mention a few. It affects 20% of human population and causing havoc as they go.

Is *staph aureus* a sexually transmitted infection?
No. It is not an STD. But a chancer. An opportunist. And can thus find its way in during sex especially if

bacteria is existing around the penis, anus and vagina area. Staph. aureus infection can affect virgins, sexually active and non-sexually active persons.

Can it be sexually transmitted?
Yes. If one partner is affected, the other can be too.

Can it affect conception and fertility?
Yes, absolutely.

Can it affect ovulation?
No, except if there is pelvic adhesion (adhesion of the reproductive organs and surrounding structures).

Can it affect period flow.
Not really except if it causes endometritis (inflammation of the womb lining) and painful periods.

It is one of the commonest infections around affecting: sperm quality, causing orchitis (inflammation of the testes) in men.

It causes in women, pelvic infection and blocked fallopian tubes.
In both genders, it may cause urine infection and infertility. In an existing pregnancy, it's a threat and may cause miscarriage or still birth.

Prevention and Treatment:
Personal hygiene is highly recommended. Please note the *s.aureus* can become resistant to treatment or become very difficult to eradicate.

Prompt and persistent treatment including treatment of sexually transmitted infections is necessary to eradicate the infection.

If you touch your nose, back passage (anus) then wash your hands thoroughly before you touch your vagina or penis. You may transmit infections if you do not follow these instructions. Keep a good skin hygiene.

36. "What is premature menopause? Is that why I am not having my periods? Can I still conceive or have my periods back?"

Normally, a woman's reproductive potential is in her age bracket 15 to 50 years. The peak reproductive age is 22 to 32 years. In general, the reproductive chances diminish as one ages. This reduction in fertility accelerates from age of 37 onwards.

However, menopause is considered as that time when a woman no longer experiences her periods for a year, at least. This is usually from age of 45-52.

Therefore, a menopause that sets in before the age of 45 is called Premature Menopause (PM). PM may lead to:

1. Lack of ovulation
2. Stoppage of periods
3. Infertility or inability to conceive
4. Sexual difficulties due to lack of vagina lubrication.
5. Reduction of female sex hormones (estrogen and progesterone) may lead to many issues like mental health decline, sleep disorders, physical health, sagging skin amongst others.

Causes of Premature Menopause
1. Genetics and inheritance from parents (See chapter one).
2. Radiation exposure say for cancer treatment.
3. Surgery to remove ovaries.
4. Exposure to toxins and chemicals.
5. Medications
6. Infection causing severe ovarian inflammation.

Solutions:
1. If you have a family history of Premature Menopause, endeavour to complete your family as soon as possible.
2. Preserve your eggs or embryo with a fertility centre sooner and use it later.
3. If all else fails, use donor eggs.
4. You may require treatment support to minimise effects of decline in sex hormones.

37. *"How can I either get pregnant when my partner is absent, difficult, or cannot even do or last a minute in bed? My time is going. Help me."*

What are your options when your reproductive potential (ability to conceive and bear children) is held down and held back by a difficult or absent partner? What would you do when the absent partner is present but he cannot last a minute in bed?

What if your partner (male or female) is manipulative, secretive, outright deceptive and or a complete time waster?

You may consider a divorce if you are married. Alternatively, you could look for a sperm or egg donor as the case may be. For erectile dysfunction, medications and other therapies could help improve erection. If the couple agrees, IUI or IVF may be the way forward.

38. *"Why do I pee so many times? In addition, it is painful. Can it affect my chances of conception? I am TTC."*

If your pee (a.k.a "urination", "wee", "number 1") is too frequent (not painful) you may have a problem likely caused by:

• Medical illnesses such as diabetes
• Too much water or any drink intake including alcohol.
• Intake of tea
• Medication or herb to control blood pressure, medications for heart disease: diuretics medications to control bleeding or firm up the uterus during child delivery or womb operations.
• Cold weather conditions.

If you have *pain* and pee too often, urge to go pee, then whether you are pregnant or not, you may be having:
• Infection of your urine system or bladder ("water infection") such as staphylococcus bacteria are common causes.
• A growth along the path of your pee. It may even be in the bladder, or kidney or tip of the pathway.
• Injury along the path of your pee.

●Recent sex may be what started your pee infection. Increased pee frequency and infection are common in pregnancy too.

Can this condition affect conception? Certainly yes. Both or either of the classes of pee may cause:
●Delay in conception.
●It may cause miscarriage
●It may cause premature delivery.
●Damage your kidney and lead to infertility.

39. ***"I have mood swings at about my ovulation and periods. Why? My breasts feel full and tingling. Am I normal?"***

Mood swings at ovulation and menstruation are known premenstrual syndrome (PMS) or disphoric disorder.

The menstrual cycle and indeed your period as well as ovulation are under control of hormones and en- zymes: FSH, LH, estrogen, progesterone and prostaglandin and many others with each one and col- lectively influencing how you feel.
Happy hormone serotonin affects your mood too.
All of these hormones and enzymes fluctuate depend- ing on the time of your cycle.
They are responsible for the mood swings you expe- rience at ovulation and period times.

They are responsible for the tingling sensation of the breasts and fullness of the breasts, abdominal swell- ing and other feelings.

As to the question of if you are well, you are well for sure. That said, if you find ovulation or periods unbearable, there are medications or preventive measure you can undertake.

40. "I am 30years old and TTC. Why am I having acne and hairs on my face? Help me."
Acne vulgaris (simple acne) or as popularly called, pimples: is in general driven by the male hormone, testosterone.

Acne is common in adolescent years when the male and female hormones are finding their balance.

At teen stage, you should know that the female hormones (estrogen, progesterone) come from the male hormone (testosterone).

However, acne may occasionally be due to a bacterium but often pimples is a result of hormone changes as mentioned above.
After the teenage years, most acnes will disappear in both girls and boys. Pregnancy may also help acne to go.

In some occasions, such as stress, pregnancy, ovulation and menstrual periods, pimples may flare up. These are "normal" and should disappear without much efforts.

However, acne that refuses to go or become troublesome has an underlying cause. Very often, such acne is due to high circulating male hormones in the woman in form of hormone imbalance. This indicates a problem in either the ovary or adrenal glands. For our purpose, the most likely cause is Polycystic Ovarian Syndrome (PCOS).

Effect: This may be responsible for the TTC and delay in conception.

Solution: The specific cause of the troublesome acne will need more investigations and treatment offered accordingly.

Chapter 13
Most Frequently Asked Questions and Comments in Fertility, Gynaecology and Andrology. Part Two.

41. *"What can I do to get pregnant with twins naturally?"*

Pregnancy occurs naturally to about 85% of couples desiring same, over a period of a year of trying to get pregnant.

Twinning or higher multiples of pregnancy is a matter of family inheritance or genetics on one hand and a matter of chance on the other hand especially for non-identical twins.

Race, such as with the Yorubas with high order of twins in Nigeria, have impact too on possibilities of having twins.

Therefore, if you marry someone with a history of twins in her or his family, from a certain place with a large likelihood of having twins, or if you are a twin yourself, your chance of having twin pregnancy is high.

Medications and nutrition may also affect your chance of having multiple pregnancies.

Lastly, medical procedures such as IVF or IUI may result in twins or multiple pregnancies.

Therefore, if you are a twin, come from a family or area of twinning, undergo medical procedures that may in the first place give you twins, then your chances are indeed huge in having twins. Nothing is guaranteed though.

So, to have twins naturally, you may need to consider your chances in view of the suggestions stated earlier. Then choose your preferred method of achieving your desire.

42. *"What can I do to prevent fibroid? Can I have my fibroid removed without surgery?"*
Fibroid is an innocent (benign, non-cancerous) growth of the uterus (womb).

The growth is very common as 80% of women will get fibroid at some stage in their life.

Risks:
Being Black or being of African descent (other races do get fibroid but not as much), obesity, high female hormone called estrogen, having had no pregnancies and lack of exercises are some circumstances that may give rise to development of fibroid.

What can you possibly do to prevent the development of fibroid?

Natural Means
•Hard as the truth may be, pregnancies are powerful breakers for the development of fibroid. While existing fibroid may grow bigger in the womb, new ones may not develop in the presence of a pregnancy.
Not having pregnancies is a risk factor.

●Logically from above breastfeeding may also prevent the growth of fibroid.

Artificial Means.
● If you are not ready for children use family planning that may suppress ovulation/estrogen/progesterone production.

●If you are done with children, consider long-term family planning that may suppress ovulation/ estrogen/progesterone production.

●Other medications are available to control growth of fibroid. Ask your doctor.

●Exercise regularly and in a structured way.

●Lose weight. Keep your weight under control or within range for your height.

●Do not consume herbs, cosmetics or medications that generate estrogen without proper supervision of a specialist.

●If you do get fibroid, pay attention: it may not trouble you. If it does trouble you, seek the help of a specialist as soon as possible.
Can fibroid re-grow after surgery? There is no guaranty that fibroid will not grow back after use of medication or after surgery.

Can you get pregnant after surgery? Yes.

43. "How do I know I am fertile?"

At any given time in a given society, about 12-15% of the reproductive age men and women are infertile. This means, over a course of a year, 85% of couples having regular sex without protection will achieve pregnancy and have a child.

It has to be said that, having your menstrual period or sign of ovulation is not a guaranteed evidence of fertility. There may be other barriers, which may affect your ability to get pregnant.

Men should not confuse ability to produce semen as proof of fertility. Semen and sperm are not the same. Normally, millions of sperm are within the fluid called semen.

Fertility doctors, Reproductive Endocrinologist and Andrologists have extensive knowledge on a range of questions to ask you and specific examinations to carry out. They will conduct comprehensive tests regarding your fertility (hormones, ultrasound, X-rays, minor surgeries and infection tests). Therefore, it is a great mistake for you to rush to do a test such as a pelvic scan or hormone assay as evidence to prove your fertility.

If you are able to prove that you are indeed fertile, what about your partner?

Conditions that may impair your fertility are many and include:

●Genetic, chromosomal, familial and inheritance disorders in your family or your spouse.

●Nutritional disorders.

●Acquired medical illnesses such as diabetes and some surgical interventions.

● Infections

●Hormone imbalance

● Tubal blockage

●Mental illnesses.

●Some medications

●Substances such as alcohol, cigarette, caffeine to mention a few.

●Above all else, your age is the most significant influence on your fertility

44. *"What is the solution to azoospermia?"*
No sperm (or azoospermia) is a serious and common issue in fertility clinics. The solution will depend on what is causing the azoospermia. In some cases, the problem can be solved through surgery or procedures to take sperm from the testes directly. If there is no ready solution, a donor sperm should be under consideration.

45. *"How can I last longer with my wife?"*

In short, I recommend you exercise regularly, jogging, aerobics of the trunk and endurance exercises. Treat any underlying illnesses including mental illness. Stop consumption of drugs, herbs and substances that disturb your performance. Alcohol comes to mind. Avoid stress. If all these are not sufficient, approach your doctor for support.

46. *"Can masturbation affect my sex life and chances of conception?"*

In my experience in dealing with clients that fall into this category, the evidence seems to support the fact that masturbating males find it difficult to relate with the female gender sexually. This is so even when the couple are married and living together. To this end, it is infertility that brings them to the clinic.

47. *"I have taken family planning injections for just 9 months. But I no longer have my periods. Can you help me get pregnant?"*

If you take family planning methods that are based on hormones be it an injection for long term or a device for a short time, your periods may be affected. If you take the tablets oral contraceptive pills for a long time, it could affect your periods. The problem is that your ovulation has been thoroughly suppressed and your period ceased. The solution is to see a fertility physician or gynaecologist to help you to ovulate. You can still conceive notwithstanding.

48. *"Can ovarian cyst stop me from getting pregnant?"*
Ovarian cysts are generally made of many types. Some are described as functional or simple and others not so or are complex. Some are cancerous especially in older age and most are not so dangerous in young age.

Some occur in young reproductive age and are often innocent cysts or functional.

Yet, perhaps the most common of them all is Poly-cystic Ovarian Disease (PCOS) accounting for up to 20% of infertility cases.

Simple and functional ovarian cyst will go away on its own and get resolved. Complex ovarian cysts require more medical attention. If your parent died of or a close relative had ovarian cancer, breast, liver, pancreas or prostate cancer, you will need to pay close attention to your ovarian cysts.

Most of the cysts do not give problems and you may not know you have cysts until you carry out an investigation or an ultrasound for other issues. Pain, pressure, irregular periods may be the symptoms of ovarian cysts depending on type, size and level of hormone meddling.

Can you get pregnant with ovarian cyst? Yes and no. It all depends on the type and if it interferes with your hormones or ovulation or blocked fallopian tubes.

49. *"Can I have positive pregnancy test and not be pregnant?"*
For good reason, an individual who is expecting to be pregnant should receive a valid pregnancy test report.

However, this is not always so. Some may ask why? And what does *chemical* pregnancy mean?
In most cases:

1. A positive pregnancy test indicates an existence of a pregnancy or recent pregnancy even if the pregnancy is recently blighted.

2. The pregnancy test strip does not answer if the pregnancy is ongoing or not. You may have delivered or miscarried the pregnancy recently.

3. The test strip does not say where the pregnancy is located. It simply says you are pregnant even if the pregnancy is ectopic.

4. Age of the pregnancy: test will be positive with blood test in first 10 days of pregnancy and 14 days using urine.

The strip simply detects a chemical (hcg) being produced by the pregnancy hence the term "chemical pregnancy". Same or similar chemical is also produced elsewhere in the body/brain at very low level either you are pregnant or not. This low level is often not a problem for pregnancy testing. If you take medication containing hcg, your pregnancy test will be positive (lasting few days though).

A valid pregnancy is one that is positive on a test strip and backed up by a practical and visible baby that is placed in the uterus/womb.

Your pregnancy test could be falsely positive:

1. If the test strip is old or damaged chemically.
2. You wait too long before reading the test.
3. If you have medical disorders such as ovarian cysts/cancer, infection of urine, brain tumors, lung, breast, liver cancers and kidney disease.
4. Molar pregnancy.
5. If you use medications such as anticonvulsant, hypnotics and tranquilizers

Can you have a negative pregnancy test and actually be pregnant? Causes of negative results:
1. Too early and too soon testing.
2. Wrong reading. Error.
3. Strip is bad, expired or damaged.
4. You are simply not pregnant.

To resolve the issue, doctors and medical specialists have other means of confirming a pregnancy.

50. *"Can you help balance my hormones?"*
The short and long answer to this question is yes. However, it depends on the cause. Some may be curable and some may not be but can be managed. Example of the illness you can manage but not cure is PCOS.

51. *"What is causing my irregular periods?"*
A few days of variation from the usual is considered normal as long as the irregularities, variations, or delays are not more than 7 days apart or length of cycle is not more than 35 days. So, the human menstrual

cycle ranges between 21 to 35 days. Some women will experience or have a cycle of 28 days. Periods often have a 3-7 day duration. Most are 5 days.

Causes of irregular periods are:
Most if not all causes are due to "Hormone Imbalance" which may be because of the following:
1. Stress (say exams, bereavements/grief, work etc.)
2. Underacting/overactive thyroid.
3.High prolactin mimicking breastfeeding. This condition has several other causes
4.Disorders such as PCOS.
5. Extreme exercising.
6. Herbs and medications.
7. Pregnancy or disorders of pregnancy.
8.Overgrown womb lining and cancers.
9. Family planning hormones.
10. Actual breast feeding.
Others are:
11. Polyps in the cervix.
12. Extremes of reproductive ages (early and late).
13. Severe weight changes, loss especially.
14. Heavy bleeding especially following a childbirth may damage the hormone producing organs and thus impairing your periods.

52. *"What steps can I do to prevent getting gynaecological diseases?*

Breast:
If you have a history of breast or ovarian cancer in your family (mother, sister, aunt siblings) or if your father has prostate cancer or close relatives have had pancreatic cancer: you are at higher risk. You may be

carrying a genetic code for breast cancer. (see Chapter One of this book)
Pay attention from early adulthood onwards. Talk to your gynaecologist immediately.

Even if you have no connection to the above mentioned cases, pay attention too. Examine your breast at least once weekly until about 70 years of age. Any lump or suspicion of a change in the breast should be an alert to pay a visit to the doctor immediately. Depending on your circumstances, the doctor may advise you to do an ultrasound or mammogram yearly or every two years.

Your *cervix* (neck of the womb) deserves a 3-yearly cancer screen unfailing. If any problem is found, a more frequent cancer screening may be suggested.

Endometrium/womb: Report any abnormal bleeding immediately to your gynaecologist.

Ovary. If you have a family history of cancer of the ovary, follow our recommendations for the breasts. If no family history, don't wait until age 65, do regular checks too. This will involve ultrasounds and other blood tests.

Infections: check for HIV, Hepatitis B and C at six monthly intervals.
Screen for HPV too. HPV causes cancer. If you are under the age of 45 years, try to get vaccinated against HPV. Chlamydia and other bacteria causes tubal blockages and infertility but no vaccination is yet

available for chlamydia. Do a check for herpes simples virus too.

53. *"My tummy is big and fat. I am not pregnant. What could be the cause?"*

Big, fat tummy is a common concern to both the victim and the clinicians that look after them. Big, fat tummy has serious implications for personal health and fertility. Commonest normal cause is pregnancy.

Other causes:
1. Nutritional causes: overeating especially fatty food and carbohydrates (sugar or starchy food). Industrially processed starch is even more risky to consume.

2. Fat deposits in abdomen and obesity due to nutritional issues, lack of exercises or genetic inheritance.

3. Medical and gynaecological illnesses in the pelvis and abdomen like:
---Fibroid
---Ovarian cysts
---Ovarian cancers
---Cancer elsewhere in the pelvis.
---Liver disorders and cancers.
---Stomach disorders including cancers
---Kidney disorders and kidney failures.
---Enlargement of the spleen.
---growths and cancers of the colon.
---Cancers from breasts, lungs, and other parts of the body.
---Heart Failure.
---Diabetes Mellitus.

4. Lack of exercises.
Regular, structured and planned physical activities /exertion.

4. Hormone Disorders
---Thyroid
---Adrenal
----Ovarian including PCOS
---Pituitary(Brain) Disorders.

5 Mental illnesses:
--depression
--Psychosis

6. Medication and herbs
--antipsychotics
--sedating antidepressants
--other medications causing weight gain.

7. Some cultural practices glorifying obesity and need to be seen as "well-fed" or "rounded".
.

Conception or fertility and general health may be affected if a big fat big tummy is not treated.

Treatment:
1. Get in touch with your medical doctor as soon as possible for screening or assessment.

2. If your big, fat tummy is a non-medical illness, then get to do 150 minutes of structured, regular, planned, exercises weekly especially abdominal exercises.

3. Pay attention to what you eat. You are what you consume.

54. *"I was abused sexually. My partner cares deeply. I don't like sex though I don't mind having kids. How can I deal with all of this?"*

Sexual abuse or misuse of a victim's reproductive system or other parts of the victim's body for sexual gratification of the abuser has serious legal, mental health and physical health concerns.

Focusing on the concerns, the following may develop in the victim of sexual abuse: let's take a look at:

Mental Health:
-- anxiety
---depression
---psychosis:
And all the consequences such as sleeplessness, self -worthlessness, suicidal ideas or attempts.
---being paranoid
---bonding difficulties
---Inability to trust
---PTSD (post-traumatic stress disorder)
---personality disorders may form and as are self in-juries.
--substance abuse (alcohol, drug misuse etc)

Gynaecology:
--Tears and injuries in vagina or beyond.
--Infection of various types: STDs, including HIV, Hepatitis B and C.
--Chronic pelvic pain (long standing pelvic pain)
---Painful and or difficult sex experiences.

---Infertility (due to infection, sex difficulties, pain, avoidance of sex, injuries to sex organs).

----Difficult childbirth.

Social:

---Difficult relationship.

---Isolation and aloofness.

Economic:

---May diminish productivity and achievement in life.

Treatment:

1. Treatment of resulting mental health issues by psychiatrist.

2. Psychological support may involve long-term psychotherapy in various forms.

3. Repair of physical injuries.

4. Medications may help you deal with the above consequences of sexual abuse.

Prevention:

1. All round the clock vigilance of the likely victim or vulnerable person to provide protection. Watchfulness of likely abuser too is required.

2. Guardian or parental education and education of likely victim or vulnerable person from as young an age as possible.

3. Teach children about sex education and uses of human body parts.

4. Victim to avoid easy material gratification or luring such as in "honey trap" manner.

5. Report of abuse or likely abuser to relevant authority (at home) and law enforcers.

6. Allow children to talk and report incidents. Never shut them down.

55. *"I have bumps below. How can I take care of it?"*
Pelvic/Vulva Skin Bumps and Rashes: Causes, Prevention and Treatment.

Causes:
1. Skin tags: which may occur naturally.
2. Folliculitis: which is inflammation of the hair follicles. May be due to too close to the skin shaving of pubic hairs.
3. Non-infectious bumps due to shaving of pubic hairs
4. Drug or chemical reaction: allergies to drugs or cosmetics.
5. Virus: human papilloma virus. (HPV)
6. Skin cancer.
7. Internal organ cancer that has spread to the skin and vulva.
8. Nerve issues: neurofibromatosis.
9.Parasites: such as worms and scabies infestation.
10. Infections: Sexually transmitted disease (STDS) such as HPV, Herpes and Non - STDS

Solutions: Prevention

1. Avoid close skin shaving. Leave about 0.5 to 1cm hair length to the skin
2. Get tested for HPV. If negative, get vaccinated
3. Watch for allergies and avoid applying substances you react to.
4. Take your personal hygiene seriously.

56. *"What causes me to bleed after sex or between my periods? Can I still conceive?"*

Bleeding after sexual intercourse or in between periods is concerning and may be due to the following:

1a. Infection of the vagina and especially of cervix (cervicitis). PID Pelvic Inflammatory Disease including sexually transmitted infection.

1. Erosion of your cervix

2. Growth:
i. Innocent (benign) growth such as polyps in the cervix and uterus.
ii. Cancer of the vagina, cancer of the cervix, endometrial cancer.

iii. Ovarian cancer or growth secreting hormones.

3. Hormone imbalance including menopause/ atrophic vaginitis (inflammation of the vagina due to lack of use of vagina or aging).

4. Injury to the reproductive track/forceful vaginal entry of the penis.

5. Medical disorders such as bleeding diseases.

6. Medications causing the body to bleed easily.

Solutions:
Vagina bleeding disorder calls for immediate visit to the gynaecologist for full assessment.

57. *"I am having persistent pain below. What is the cause? Will I be able to conceive?"*
Persistent pelvic pain could be due to many causes such as endometriosis, pelvic infection, fibroid, pelvic congestion syndrome, urinary bladder and kidney infection, ovarian cysts, irritable bowel amongst others. The way forward is to undergo a check to find the cause. Conception is possible depending on each particular circumstance.

58. *"What treatment do you have for low sperm count?*
Low sperm count could be due to a varied number of causes. Some may be genetic. Others may be due to your behavior and what you eat or what you failed to eat. The first step is to find the likely cause and remove such hindrances. If no specific cause is detected, my approach is to boost the sperm with drugs and herbs. I also advise on need for change in nutrition and lifestyle. Do exercise regularly. Avoid heating up the testes.

59. *"Help me calculate my ovulation day"*
When did my egg break? How do I know my ovulation time and fertile time? Can I time my ovulation? How do I know if I have ovulated? These and similar questions are what we are frequently asked.

Either you have regular or irregular periods, your ovulation will occur about 14 days before the first day of your next menstrual period. Put in another way, you ovulated 14 days ago if your period started today. Examples: In a 28-day cycle, ovulation is on day 14. In 21-day cycle, ovulation is on Day 7.

You can plan your pregnancy around this fact.

60. *"I had sex 4 days after my period, can I get pregnant?"*

This is likely if your menstrual cycle is 21days and your period lasted 3 days. Therefore, you may ovulate 4 days after your period (day 7 of your cycle) and then get pregnant.

61. *How much is your IVF?*

At least in our practice, IVF is individualized. No two persons or couples are the same. Besides, market forces change rapidly especially in view of unstable currency and inflation. In addition, providing a fixed fee may short-change the consumer as the procedure consumes more human and material resources along the way. Above all, our practice is to evaluate the patient as the couple or individual may not require IVF to get pregnant. Committing to a specific IVF fee is therefore not feasible considering the unforeseeable determinants of life today

62. *How much is your IUI?*

The answer is much the same as for IVF. Nothing is fixed until full evaluation is done.

63. I don't like sex and I find sex painful. How can I get pregnant?

Painful sex or difficult sex is called dyspareunia. What causes it?

1. Pain on entry into Vagina
Penis entry into vagina can be difficult because you have:

a) Poor lubrication
b) Injury/trauma, female circumcision, childbirth, obstructive hymen: (hymen is a thing tissue covering the vagina).
c) Infection such as herpes and urine infection, PID
d) Physical abnormality from birth
e) Mismatch of sizes of sexual organs. That is, if you have small vagina and the penis is big, you could have painful sex.
(f) Vaginismus (defined as involuntary spasms of the muscles of the vaginal wall which can make penile penetration of vaginal painful): this can be due to:
a) Anxiety, stress, depression
b) Fear
c) Religious or cultural conditioning
d) Poor foreplay
e) Infection
f) Dryness of vagina

2. Deep sexual pain can be due to:
a) Previous surgical operations in pelvis including hysterectomy,
b) Pelvic diseases such as prolapse and infections.
3. Sexual abuse could lead to difficult sexual experience.

Can you conceive with painful sex? Natural conception may be difficult with each of these conditions and may thus require that the illnesses be treated or assisted conception may be considered. (see Chapter on assisted conception)

Solutions: The solution is to address the cause(s) as outlined above.

You may need the support of a gynaecologist and fertility specialist to help you.
The way out of this difficult situation could be IUI, IVF or surrogacy.

64. *"I have not seen my period for a year and I am not pregnant. Why Dr? What can I do? I want my own kids."*
Amenorrhoea is absence of menstrual periods (unlike menstrual periods appearing after more than 35 days which is called oligomenorrhoea) for more than 6 months at a go.

This condition may have serious effects on your fertility and conception.

Can fertility and or conception be affected? Yes. Others may not. So, get to see your physician for assessment.

65. *"Why am I not getting pregnant?"*
"Why am I not getting pregnant?"
This is perhaps one of our commonest FAQs Let's look at some reasons for fertility delays.

In men:
1. Sperm abnormalities is a key factor.
2. Erectile dysfunction is common.
3. Diseases of the sperm ejaculatory tube like blockage.
4. Hostile environment to sperm (heat, infections sperm antibodies etc.)
5. Infection anywhere in the sperm's way.
6. Hormone imbalance.
7. Others: Medical illnesses, genetic, blood disorders etc.
8. Surgery including family planning.
9.Substance misuse (cannabis, alcohol, nicotine for examples).
10. Mental health issues.

Common causes to both male and female: Long distance relationship and lack of exercise

In women.
1. Hormone imbalance (loads of causes such as PCOS, high prolactin).
2. Lack of ovulation.
3. Diseases of the tube (tubal blockage, water and pus collection in tubes)
4. Diseases of the womb (infection, large fibroids, blocked endometrial space)
5. Diseases of the cervix (weak cervix, hostile mucus, antibodies against sperm).
6. Diseases of the vagina (poor lubrication to sex, infection, pain etc.)
7. Diseases of the ovaries.
8. Mental health issues: depression, anxiety.

9. Stress.
10. Medical diseases---uncontrolled diabetes.
11. Others such as endometriosis.
12. Aging: a crucial factor.
13. Medications & surgery including family planning.
14. Substance misuse (alcohol, nicotine etc.)

66. *"Can staphylococcus be transmitted sexually?"*
Strictly, s. aureus is not considered a sexually transmitted infection. However, once a partner is affected, the other may get the infection through sex.

67. *"Can staphylococcus block my tubes?"*
Yes.

68. *"Why am I having breast discharge?"*
Causes in women. (Causes in men are slightly different but in general similar to women). Medications: for example: certain sedatives, antipsychotics and high blood pressure medicines. Opioid such as morphine use. Herbal additions, including anise seed. Oral contraceptive pills or birth control pills may also be blamable. A pituitary tumor in the brain (prolactinoma) or other disorder of the pituitary organ.

Underactive thyroid otherwise known as hypothyroidism. Long standing kidney disease may be responsible too. Excessive breast stimulation during sexual activity and nipple manipulation or prolonged clothing that stimulates the nipples. Nerve damage to the chest wall from chest surgery, burns or other chest injuries. Injury to spinal cord. Stressful conditions.

Pregnancy: miscarried or not. These are the likely causes of your nipple discharge.

69. *"I do not ovulate. Can you help me ovulate?"*

Causes of lack of ovulation: Few years after onset on periods, ovulation may be erratic as the hormones settle down and later stabilise. At menopause and few years before the closure of reproductive potential, ovulation becomes erratic too just as the hormones fluctuate. Premature ovarian failure or dysfunction, which may occur at any age, may disturb ovulation. Hormone imbalance issues such as high prolactin. Ovarian disorders such as PCOS especially. Menstrual disorders such as endometriosis may impair egg pickup even if there is ovulation. Absence of ovaries from birth. Absence or reduced function of ovaries due to surgery. Medications and family planning hormones may suppress ovulation. Treatments or exposure to chemotherapy or radiotherapy may impair the ovaries. Stress, depression or mental health issues and their medications may suppress ovulation. Other illnesses affecting the brain, thyroid, adrenals, kidney and liver may impair the function of your reproductive hormones.

Infection such as mumps in childhood or other times and adult infection such as pelvic inflammatory disease (PID) may cost you ovulation. Genetic/chromosomal disorders could make ovulation difficult.

70. *"Can you help open my blocked tubes?"*

Tubes that are blocked can be opened up. There are various ways of opening depending on the cause in each particular case.

71. *"My progesterone is low. I want to raise it. What can I use?"*

Progesterone is a key hormone in women's wellbeing and crucial to their ability to bear children.

At any given moment, men and women do have varying levels of progesterone. However, different amounts of progesterone are required at different times in order for the reproductive system to function well. Example: the amount of progesterone required at fertilization is different from the quantity needed to sustain pregnancy.

What causes low progesterone? Some are mentioned here:

1. PCOS
2. Lack of ovulation
3. Post ovulation failure of progesterone- secreting organ (corpus luteum).
4. Anti-progesterone medications and herbs.
5. Aging and extremes of reproductive ages.
.

Solution: You cannot handle this on your own.

72. *"What causes blighted ovum? Can I still have children of my own?"*

1. Abnormalities of the foetus. (baby in the womb) itself such as chromosomal abnormalities.
2. Infections of the womb.
3. Genetic abnormalities of either or both parents.
4. Blood or hormone disorders in the mother.

5. Toxic uterine environment of any cause (chemicals including herbals; drugs and substances such as alcohol, cigarettes consumption) that stiffen growth.
6. Medical illnesses such as diabetes, in the mother.

Most causes of blighted ovum as listed above are also responsible for miscarriages.

7. Age of the mother and father matters. The older the mother, the more the risk of miscarriage and blighted ovum due to hormone disorders, structural abnormalities of the womb or chromosomal errors occurring in the embryo and eggs. The fathers who are above 65 years may also carry damaged sperms that leads to blighted ovum and miscarriage.
8. For miscarriage specifically, even if everything else is good, neck of the womb weakness may cause pregnancy loss among other causes. Included in this list is structural uterine oddities.

73. *"Can I remove my fibroid without surgery"?*
Fibroid may sometimes be removed without the normal surgical procedures. Some inventions using high intensity sound, may help in this respect. That said, majority of fibroids are removed by surgery if removal is necessary in the first instance.

74. *"Why I am having repeated pelvic infections?"*
Pelvic Inflammatory Disease (PID) is primarily due to infection that affects pelvic reproductive organs. The infection leads to inflammation (bad odour, pain, swelling, changes in colour and heat generation). That is why it is called "inflammation."

The infection may be a sexually transmitted disease such as gonorrhoea, Chlamydia and many other sexually related infections. Pelvic infections may not be sexually transmitted. It may have been a contamination from your skin and areas around your vagina and anus. Example of this is Staphylococcus & E.coli.
Viruses & parasites may cause PID Pelvic Inflammatory Disease too. If you have poor personal hygiene, such as leaving vaginal pads/tampons in place for too long, you may get pelvic infections. Yeasts may cause PID.

Complications/effects: Offensive/bad odour from vaginal discharge, abdominal pain, painful periods painful sex are some hitches from pelvic infections. Fever may occur. When problems occur, the ovary may suffer inflammation as may the rest of the pelvic organs and abdomen. The fallopian tubes may be blocked or have a collection of water or pus in them. The womb may suffer from inflammation (as endometritis). The most serious complications from the ertility standpoint are tubal blockages, ovarian abscess, infertility and miscarriages. Remember that sexual partners catch the infections. Therefore, his sperm may not work well because of the contaminations. The partner will therefore need treatment for infection. PID or pelvic infection generally is not friendly to pregnancy and may affect the baby. *Prevention*: Your personal hygiene matters greatly. Stick to a single sexual partner or use condoms, provided your sexual partner sticks with only yourself. Treat suspected PID promptly. Screen your sexual partner for infections before sex. Your partner should get treatment at the same time as you.

75. *"I am diagnosed with uterine adhesions. Can I still be pregnant?"*

Pregnancy is certainly possible after treatment of the adhesions.

76. *"I have had many miscarriages. My doctor said I have cervical incompetence. What can I do? Can you help me?"*

Causes of miscarriage:

1. Abnormalities of the foetus (baby in the womb) itself such as chromosomal abnormalities.

2. Infections of the womb.

3. Genetic abnormalities of either or both parents.

4. Blood or hormone disorders in the mother.

5. Toxic uterine environment of any cause (chemicals including herbals; drugs and substances such as alcohol, cigarettes consumption) that stiffen growth.

6. Medical illnesses such as diabetes, in the mother.

7. Age of the mother and father matters. The older the mother, the more the risk of miscarriage due to hormone disorders, structural abnormalities of the womb or chromosomal errors occurring in the children. The fathers who are above 65 years may also negatively impact pregnancy.

.
8. For miscarriage specifically, even if everything else is good, neck of the womb weakness may cause pregnancy loss amongst other causes. This weakness of the neck of the womb is called *cervical incompetence.* Often, cervical incompetence is due to natural weakness, operations like dilatation and curettage (D & C) tears amongst others.

77. *"Why am I itching so much down below?"*

Itching is a common symptom in women and it can be troublesome. Sometimes we see itching in men too in pelvic areas.

Most common causes are thrush or fungi that comes with thick whitish vaginal discharge. Thrush is also called candidiasis. It may be connected with pregnancy and diabetes or comes occurring on its own. Some parasites, bacteria or viruses (herpes) non-STD or STD infections may also cause vaginal or vulva itching. In elderly women, long-standing itching called *lichen sclerosus et atrophicus,* not related to infection may occur. Anxiety and other medical disorders may cause itching too.

78. *"I am told I have retroverted uterus. Is that why I find it difficult to conceive?"*

A uterus (womb) turned backwards is called a retroverted uterus. It means a womb that is turned backwards instead of forward. Some women may experience symptoms including painful sex. Most often, a retroverted uterus won't cause any problem during pregnancy. Note that about 10-20% of women suffer from this problem of a retroverted uterus. This condition on its own will not stop you from conceiving. Causes: It could be normal or due to genetics. Some cases are caused by pelvic surgery, pelvic adhesions, endometriosis, fibroids, pelvic inflammatory disease, or childbirth.

79. *"I have delayed ejaculation. What can I use?"*
Causes:

a. Priapism (erection that fails to relax and remain firm and painful. Unwanted persistent painful erection).

b. No semen available to ejaculate.

c. Excessive recent sexual activities.

d. Herbs & drugs e.g antidepressants.

e. Poor lubrication of vagina.

f. Poor sensation of the penis e.g. diabetes.

g. Nerve injury locally or at spinal cord.

i. Exhaustion/stress.

j. Blood disorders e.g. sickle cell.

If you don't seem to ejaculate at all, it may mean that the semen is going elsewhere such as backwards into the urinary bladder. This condition is called *retrograde ejaculation*.

80. *"I am a 48 year old woman. Why am I sweating so much? I am TTC and I last had my period 3 months ago. Can you help me?"*
Considering the age and symptoms of sweating, it appears this condition is menopause or early phase of going into menopause. This condition comes with

hormone imbalance. Symptoms could include sweating, internal heat, irregular periods, considerably reduced fertility, irritability, poor vaginal lubrication, poor sleep amongst others. It is not old women's tales. The victims and sufferers are neither mentally unwell nor are they witches as some may want us believe. For some women, new biotechnology method has enabled us to delay menopause or renew their fertility in ovarian rejuvenation procedure that may also give a chance of conception. We do engage in ovarian rejuvenation and have restored hope to some of our clients.

81. *"In which fertility treatment area is physical exercise going to help me? Can exercise and Relaxation help me?"*
The long and short answer is yes. Regular, structured and planned exercises can improve fertility, decrease weight, improve sex, prevent up to 13 cancers including breast and endometrial cancers. In men, exercises improve stamina, prevent prostate cancer, and increase sperm quality. Exercises calm the nerves and improve depression.

82. *How will I know if I am pregnant? What medication should I take or avoid?*
Early pregnancy can seem like feverish conditions & feeling of being unwell like malaria, tired or have cold-like illness. In almost all persons, you will miss your period. You may have nausea and vomiting. Go do a pregnancy test as soon as possible. Take no medication, alcohol, substances or herbs until pregnancy is confirmed or excluded by blood/urine test or via

ultrasound scan if you are to avoid damaging the baby and pregnancy. Even when your pregnancy is confirmed by ultrasound, in the first two months, avoid almost all drug preparations except well tested drugs and ones that are trusted to be safe in pregnancy. Avoid anti-malaria. Chloroquine with piriton or with Phenergan are safe throughout pregnancy. Ensure you go to a competent doctor and preferably a gynaecologist as soon as you discover that you are pregnant.

83. *"Can I get pregnant with endometriosis?*

Getting pregnant with endometriosis is possible. The chances of getting pregnant can be by natural means or with the help of fertility medicine or fertility doctors.

Endometriosis is a serious, painful and frequently energy-sapping, gynaecological illness. Infertility is often a hurdle as part of this disorder.

Origin of endometriosis: no one knows for sure. There are many theories about what causes endometriosis. One thing is sure: womb lining is found where they should not be. Example: They are found in the fallopian tubes, ovaries, abdomen and even in the chest.

How it affects health: painful period is common. Infertility is a well-known complication. Victims suffer a lot.

Treatment options:
1. Control of pain by various classes of medications.
2. Surgery to remove parts of the endometriotic tissues and to free affected organs.

146

3. Assisted conception if complications prevent getting pregnant naturally.
4. Medications to regulate the effect of or defer menstruation.
5. Combination of any or all of the above

Miscellaneous Lists

I. A list of some common sexually transmitted diseases (STD) that may kill you, affect your fertility, or affect the quality of your life. Alternatively, they may seriously affect your newborn child.

Viruses
Hepatitis B
Hepatitis C
Herpes 1 (cold sore) and *Type 2*. Type 2 occurs in the pelvic area. Herpes can affect the eyes, hand (as whitlow) and any part of the skin. Type 1 and 2 can be deadly if it became widespread or got to the blood of victims. Herpes can cause inflammation of the brain in young or older persons. A newborn is at high risk of serious illness such as brain inflammation (meningitis) if infected by herpes. Newborn has low immunity to defend the body. If you have cold sore or sore in any part of your body, do not touch or kiss a new baby. Do not let anyone kiss or touch your new baby if you are unsure of his or her herpes status. Herpes can kill an adult if the immunity is low or it becomes widespread during surgery. Other viruses:
Human Immunodeficiency Virus (HIV)
Human Papilloma Virus (HPV)
Acquired Immune Deficiency Syndrome (AIDS) from HIV

Bacteria
Chlamydia
Gonorrhoea
Lyphogranuloma venerum (Caused by unique strains of chlamydia).
Syphilis

148

Fungus:
Thrush/Candidiasis

Parasite
Trichomoniasis
Scabies

Sexually transmitted infections such as gonorrhoea and chlamydia are major causes of pelvic inflammatory disease (PID) and infertility in women and a threat to a newborn child

II. Common Non-STD or non-classic STD that may still affect your fertility.

Staphylococcus aureus
E.coli
Ureaplasma urealyticum

III. Common Fertility Tests (depending on individual person's circumstances)

For women
Ultrasound
Hormone profile
Infection screen
Tubal patency (by X-Ray or by Laparoscopy) test

For men
Seminal Fluid Analysis and culture
Hormone profile
Infection screen (as listed above)

IV. Tests you should consider before you form a sexual relationship, marriage, or undergo childbearing

Genetic
Genotype (such as sickle cell disease, cyctic fibrosis)
Any other familial or inherited /genetic diseases

Infection screen
As listed under STD and Non-STD as listed above
Mental health assessment
Look at the family tree and background. Ask specific questions and make your own discrete inquiries.

V. Common Fertility Tests You Should Consider.
As above listed plus the following:

Drug screen
Alcohol
Cannabis
Nicotine
Cocaine and any other drug you may suspect.

Other tests
Blood group

VI. Desirable Sperm Qualities
Good sperm count
Good morphology
Good motility

Book by the same author

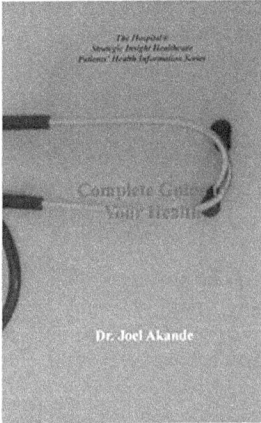

About the Book. *Complete Guide to Your Health* is a medical compendium purposely written in plain English and devoid of complicated medical jargon. The purpose is to provide the readers with comprehensive guide to total health, emphasising simple-to-adopt, common sense measures to safeguard health.

Contact of the author:
www.the-hospitals.com
managementlease@gmail.com

References

1. Sandstead HH. Understanding zinc: recent observations and interpretations. J Lab Clin Med 1994;124:322-7. [PubMed abstract]

2. Institute of Medicine, Food and Nutrition Board. Dietary Reference Intakes for Vitamin A, Vitamin K, Arsenic, Boron, Chromium, Copper, Iodine, Iron, Manganese, Molybdenum, Nickel, Silicon, Vanadium, and Zinc external link disclaimer. Washington, DC: National Academy Press, 2001.

3. National Institute of Health: https://ods.od.nih.gov/factsheets/Zinc-HealthProfessional/#en1

4. Favier AE. Biol Trace Elem Res. 1992 Jan-Mar; 32:363-82.

5. FAO: Role of vitamin B12 in human metabolic processes. http://www.fao.org/3/Y2809E/y2809e0b.htm

6. Saleem Ali Banihani. Vitamin B12 and Semen Quality. Biomolecules. 2017 Jun; 7(2): 42.

7. Mackey A, Davis S, Gregory J. Vitamin B6. In: Shils M, Shike M, Ross A, Caballero B, Cousins R, eds. Modern Nutrition in Health and Disease. 10th ed. Baltimore, MD: Lippincott Williams & Wilkins; 2005.

8. C. J. Thaler. Folate Metabolism and Human Reproduction. Geburtshilfe Frauenheilkd. 2014 Sep; 74(9): 845–851. https://www.ncbi.nlm.nih.gov/pmc/articles/PMC4175124/

9. National Institute of Health. https://ods.od.nih.gov/factsheets/Folate-HealthProfessional/

10. FAO. Folate and folic acid. http://www.fao.org/3/Y2809E/y2809e0a.htm#TopOfPage

11. https://www.webmd.com/vitamins/ai/ingredientmono-965/thiamine-vitamin-b1

12. FAO: Thiamin, riboflavin, niacin, vitamin B6, pantothenic acid and biotin. http://www.fao.org/3/Y2809E/y2809e09.htm#TopOfPage

13. Nutrition and Metabolic Insights. First Published March 15, 2017. https://doi.org/10.1177/1178638817693824

14. Basil V. Peechakara; Mohit Gupta. Vitamin B2 (Riboflavin). Treasure Island (FL): StatPearls Publishing; 2019 Jan-. https://www.ncbi.nlm.nih.gov/books/NBK525977/

15. https://www.webmd.com/diet/niacin-deficiency-symptoms-and-treatments#1

16. Adrian C Williams and Lisa J Hill. Nicotinamide's Ups and Downs: Consequences for Fertility, Development, Longevity and Diseases of Poverty and Affluence.Int J Tryptophan Res. 2018; 11: 1178646918802289. https://www.ncbi.nlm.nih.gov/pmc/articles/PMC6178124/

17. Margaret Clagett-Dame1and Danielle Knutson. Vitamin A in Reproduction and Development. Nutrients. 2011 Apr; 3(4): 385–428. https://www.ncbi.nlm.nih.gov/pmc/articles/PMC3257687/

18. FAO. Role of vitamin A in human metabolic processes. http://www.fao.org/3/Y2809E/y2809e0d.htm#TopOfPage

19. FAO. Vitamin C. http://www.fao.org/3/Y2809E/y2809e0c.htm#TopOfPage

20. Luck MR, Jeyaseelan I, Scholes RA. Ascorbic acid and fertility. Biol Reprod. 1995 Feb;52(2):262-6.

21. National Institute of Health. Vitamin C. https://ods.od.nih.gov/factsheets/VitaminC-HealthProfessional/

22. Crha I, Hrubá D, Ventruba P, Fiala J, Totusek J, Visnová H. Ascorbic acid and infertility treatment. Cent Eur J Public Health. 2003 Jun;11(2):63-7. https://www.ncbi.nlm.nih.gov/pubmed/12884545

23. Hirofumi Henmi et al. Effects of ascorbic acid supplementation on serum progesterone levels in patients with a luteal phase defect. Fert-Sterility. August 2003Volume 80, Issue 2, Pages 459–461. https://www.fertstert.org/article/S0015-0282(03)00657-5/fulltext

24. Grzechocinska B, Dabrowski FA, Cyganek A, Wielgos M. The role of vitamin D in impaired fertility treatment. Neuro Endocrinol Lett. 2013;34(8):756-62. https://www.ncbi.nlm.nih.gov/pubmed/24522025

25. Daniels LA. Selenium metabolism and bioavailability. Biol Trace Elem Res. 1996 Sep;54(3):185-99. https://www.ncbi.nlm.nih.gov/pubmed/8909692

26. Mistry HD, Broughton Pipkin F, Redman CW, Poston L. Selenium in reproductive health. Am J Obstet Gynecol. 2012 Jan;206(1):21-30. doi: 10.1016/j.ajog.2011.07.034. Epub 2011 Jul 29. https://www.ncbi.nlm.nih.gov/pubmed/21963101

27. Izhar Hyder Qazi et al. Selenium, Selenoproteins, and Female Reproduction: A Review. Molecules. 2018 Dec; 23(12): 3053. https://www.ncbi.nlm.nih.gov/pmc/articles/PMC6321086/

28. Pal A. Role of Copper and Selenium in Reproductive Biology: A Brief Update. Pal, Biochem Pharmacol (Los Angel) 2015, 4:4. DOI: 10.4173/2167-0501.1000181

29. Meseguer M et al. The human sperm glutathione system: a key role in male fertility and successful cryopreservation. Drug Metab Lett. 2007 Apr;1(2):121-6. https://www.ncbi.nlm.nih.gov/pubmed/19356030

30. Oyewopo Adeoye et al. Review on the role of glutathione on oxidative stress and infertility. JBRA Assist Reprod. 2018 Jan-Mar; 22(1): 61–66. https://www.ncbi.nlm.nih.gov/pmc/articles/PMC5844662/

31 What foods are high in glutathione? https://www.webmd.com/cold-and-flu/qa/what-foods-are-high-in-glutathione

32. Joseph Pizzorno. Glutathione! Integr Med (Encinitas). 2014 Feb; 13(1): 8–12. https://www.ncbi.nlm.nih.gov/pmc/articles/PMC4684116/

33. What you should know about Glutathione. https://duramental.de/en/was-sie-ueber-glutathion-wissen-sollten/

34. Goral S. Levocarnitine and muscle metabolism in patients with end-stage renal disease. J Ren Nutr. 1998 Jul;8(3):118-21. https://www.ncbi.nlm.nih.gov/pubmed/9724499

35. Judith L Flanagan, Peter A Simmons, Joseph Vehige, Mark DP Willcox & Qian Garrett . Role of carnitine in disease. Nutrition & Metabolismvolume 7, Article number: 30 (2010). https://nutritionandmetabolism.biomedcentral.com/articles/10.1186/1743-7075-7-30

36. Ashok Agarwal,, Pallav Sengupta, and Damayanthi Durairajanayagam. Role of L-carnitine in female infertility. Reprod Biol Endocrinol. 2018; 16: 5. doi: 10.1186/s12958-018-0323-4

37. A Agarwal, Tamer M Said. Carnitines and male infertility. Reproductive Biomedicine Online. DOI: https://doi.org/10.1016/S1472-6483(10)60920-0

38. National Institute of Health: Carnitine. https://ods.od.nih.gov/factsheets/Carnitine-HealthProfessional/

39. Zhe Xu et al. Coenzyme Q10 Improves Lipid Metabolism and Ameliorates Obesity by Regulating CaMKII-Mediated PDE4 Inhibition.

40. Yangying Xu. Pretreatment with coenzyme Q10 improves ovarian response and embryo quality in low-prognosis young women with decreased ovarian reserve: a randomized controlled trial Reprod Biol Endocrinol. 2018; 16: 29. doi: 10.1186/s12958-018-0343-0. https://www.ncbi.nlm.nih.gov/pmc/articles/PMC5870379/

41. Assaf Ben-Meir et al. Coenzyme Q10 restores oocyte mitochondrial function and fertility during reproductive aging. Aging Cell. 2015 Oct; 14(5): 887–895. doi: 10.1111/acel.12368. https://www.ncbi.nlm.nih.gov/pmc/articles/PMC4568976/

42. Yaakov Bentov, M.D., and Robert F. Casper, M.D. The aging oocyte—can mitochondrial function be improved?. Fert-Ster. Volume 99, Issue 1, Pages 18–22. https://www.fertstert.org/article/S0015-0282(12)02443-0/fulltext

43. WebMD. Coenzyme Q10: CoQ10. https://www.webmd.com/diet/supplement-guide-coenzymeq10-coq10#1

44..L.Palmquist. Omega-3 Fatty Acids in Metabolism, Health, and Nutrition and for Modified Animal Product Foods. Omega-3 Fatty Acids in

Metabolism, Health, and Nutrition and for Modified Animal Product Foods.

45. Mohammad Reza Safarinejad and Shiva Safarinejad. The roles of omega-3 and omega-6 fatty acids in idiopathic male infertility. Asian J Androl. 2012 Jul; 14(4): 514–515. doi: 10.1038/aja.2012.46.

46. Hosseini B et al. The Effect of Omega-3 Fatty Acids, EPA, and/or DHA on Male Infertility: A Systematic Review and Meta-analysis. J Diet Suppl. 2019;16(2):245-256. doi: 10.1080/19390211.2018.1431753. Epub 2018 Feb 16. https://www.ncbi.nlm.nih.gov/pubmed/29451828

47. How Much Omega-3 Should You Take Per Day? https://www.health-line.com/nutrition/how-much-omega-3

48 National Institute of Health: Omega-3 Fatty Acids. https://ods.od.nih.gov/factsheets/Omega3FattyAcids-Consumer/

49. Recommended Dietary Allowances: 10th Edition (1989). Page 52. National Academic Press. ISBN 978-0-309-04041-9 | DOI 10.17226/1349

50. B Buzadzic et al. New insights into male (in)fertility: the importance of NO. Br J Pharmacol. 2015 Mar; 172(6): 1455–1467.

51. van Die MD, Burger HG, Teede HJ, Bone KM. Vitex agnus-castus extracts for female reproductive disorders: a systematic review of clinical trials. Planta Med. 2013 May;79(7):562-75. doi: 10.1055/s-0032-1327831. Epub 2012 Nov 7.

52. Niroumand MC, Heydarpour F, Farzaei MH. Pharmacological and therapeutic effects of Vitex agnus-castus L.: A review. Phcog Rev [serial online] 2018 [cited 2019 Sep 18];12:103-14. Available from: http://www.phcogrev.com/text.asp?2018/12/23/103/232188

53. Babu PS, Stanely Mainzen Prince P. Antihyperglycaemic and antioxidant effect of hyponidd, an ayurvedic herbomineral formulation in streptozotocin-induced diabetic rats. J Pharm Pharmacol. 2004 Nov;56(11):1435-42.

54. Sridharan K, Mohan R, Ramaratnam S, Panneerselvam D. Ayurvedic treatments for diabetes mellitus. Cochrane Database Syst Rev. 2011 Dec 7;(12):CD008288. doi: 10.1002/14651858.CD008288.pub2.

55. M. Ayyanar and S. Ignacimuthu , 2008. Pharmacological Actions of Cassia auriculata L. and Cissus quadrangularis Wall.: A Short Review. Journal of Pharmacology and Toxicology, 3: 213-221. https://scial-ert.net/abstract/?doi=jpt.2008.213.221

56.   Sunday Odunke Nduka. Herb drug interaction: effect of Manix® on pharmacokinetic parameters of pefloxacin in rat model. Asian Pac J Trop Biomed. 2014 May; 4(Suppl 1): S413–S416. doi: 10.12980/APJTB.4.2014C400 https://www.ncbi.nlm.nih.gov/pmc/arti-cles/PMC4025296/ .

57. Kehinde Habeeb Tijani , K Adegoke, A A Oluwole, J Ogunlewe. The role of manix in the management of idiopathic oligospermia. A pilot study at the Lagos University Teaching Hospital Nigerian quarterly journal of hospital medicine 18(3):142-4 · July 2008.

58. Rajeev Kumar et al. Herbo-mineral supplementation in men with idio-pathic oligoasthenoteratospermia : A double blind randomized placebo-controlled trial. Indian J Urol. 2011 Jul-Sep; 27(3): 357–362. doi: 10.4103/0970-1591.85440.

59. Anthony Jide Afolayan, Musa Toyin. Erectile Dysfunction Manage-ment Options in Nigeria. Journal of Sexual Medicine. Volume6, Issue. April 2009 Pages 1090-1102. https://doi.org/10.1111/j.1743-6109.2008.01064.x

60. Sabna Kotta, Shahid H. Ansari,1 and Javed Ali. Exploring scientifi-cally proven herbal aphrodisiacs. Pharmacogn Rev. 2013 Jan-Jun; 7(13): 1–10. doi: 10.4103/0973-7847.112832.
https://www.ncbi.nlm.nih.gov/pmc/articles/PMC3731873/

61. Al-Yahya AA, Al-Majed AA, Al-Bekairi AM, Al-Shabanah OA, Qureshi S. Studies on the reproductive, cytological and biochemical tox-icity of Ginkgo Biloba in Swiss albino mice. J Ethnopharmacol. 2006 Sep 19;107(2):222-8. Epub 2006 Mar 27. https://www.ncbi.nlm.nih.gov/pub-med/16624513

62. Wolfgang Elmar Paulus et al. Application of ginkgo biloba in assisted reproduction therapy Fert-SterVol. 78, No. 3, Suppl. 1, September 2002

63. Matthias Unger (2013) Pharmacokinetic drug interactions involving Ginkgo biloba, Drug Metabolism Reviews, 45:3, 353-385, DOI: 10.3109/03602532.2013.815200

64. Asmaa Ibrahim Ahmed, Noha N. Lasheen,, and Khaled Mohamed El-Zawahry Ginkgo Biloba Ameliorates Subfertility Induced by Testicular Ischemia/Reperfusion Injury in Adult Wistar Rats: A Possible New Mitochondrial Mechanism. Oxid Med Cell Longev. 2016; 2016: 6959274. doi: 10.1155/2016/6959274

65. Leonardo Toshio Oshio, Teixeira Ribeiro Claudia Cristina, Macedo Marques Renato, Martha de Oliveira Guerra. Effect of Ginkgo biloba extract on sperm quality, serum testosterone concentration and histometric analysis of testes from adult Wistar rats. DOI: 10.5897/JMPR2015.5730

66. https://www.drugs.com/npp/lady-s-mantle.html

67 NIH. Evening Primrose Oil. https://nccih.nih.gov/health/eveningprimrose

68. Rahil Jannatifar, Kazem Parivar, Nasim Hayati Roodbari & Mohammad Hossein Nasr-Esfahani. Effects of N-acetyl-cysteine supplementation on sperm quality, chromatin integrity and level of oxidative stress in infertile men. Reproductive Biology and Endocrinologyvolume 17, Article number: 24 (2019)

69. M.A. Bedaiwy, A. RezkH. Al Inany, T. Falcone. N-acetyl cystein improves pregnancy rate in long standing unexplained infertility: A novel mechanism of ovulation induction. Volume 82, Supplement 2, Page S228. DOI: https://doi.org/10.1016/j.fertnstert.2004.07.604

70 Int J Endocrinol. 2016; 2016: 9537632.. Myoinositol as a Safe and Alternative Approach in the Treatment of Infertile PCOS Women: A German Observational Study.

71. Regidor PA, Schindler AE, Lesoine B3, Druckman R Management of women with PCOS using myo-inositol and folic acid. New clinical data

and review of the literature. Horm Mol Biol Clin Investig. 2018 Mar 2;34(2). doi: 10.1515/hmbci-2017-0067.

72. Norbert Gleichercorresponding and David H Barad. Dehydroepiandrosterone (DHEA) supplementation in diminished ovarian reserve (DOR). Reprod Biol Endocrinol. 2011; 9: 67.
https://www.ncbi.nlm.nih.gov/pmc/articles/PMC3112409/

73. Yilmaz N, Uygur D, Inal H, Gorkem U, Cicek N, Mollamahmutoglu L. Dehydroepiandrosterone supplementation improves predictive markers for diminished ovarian reserve: serum AMH, inhibin B and antral follicle count. Eur J Obstet Gynecol Reprod Biol. 2013 Jul;169(2):257-60. doi: 10.1016/j.ejogrb.2013.04.003. Epub 2013 May 9.
https://www.ncbi.nlm.nih.gov/pubmed/23664458

74. Siti Syairah Mohd Mutalip,,Sharaniza Ab-Rahim, and Mohd Hamim Rajikin. Vitamin E as an Antioxidant in Female Reproductive Health. Antioxidants (Basel). 2018 Feb; 7(2): 22. doi: 10.3390/antiox7020022.

75. Liu S, Shi L, Wang T, Shi J. Effect of low-dose dexamethasone on patients with elevated early follicular phase progesterone level and pregnancy outcomes in IVF-ET treatment: A randomized controlled clinical trial [published online July 27, 2018]. Clin Endocrinol (Oxf). doi: 10.1111/cen.13824. https://onlinelibrary.wiley.com/doi/pdf/10.1111/cen.13824

76. Benoit B. N'guessan et al. In Vitro Antioxidant Potential and Effect of a Glutathione-Enhancer Dietary Supplement on Selected Rat Liver Cytochrome P450 Enzyme Activity. Evid Based Complement Alternat Med. 2018; 2018: 7462839. https://www.ncbi.nlm.nih.gov/pmc/articles/PMC5994258/

78. Hiromi Sawamur. Dietary intake of high-dose biotin inhibits spermatogenesis in young rats. Congenital Anomalies 2015; 55, 31–36.

79. Guruprasad Kalthur et al. Supplementation of biotin to sperm preparation medium increases the motility and longevity in cryopreserved human spermatozoa. J Assist Reprod Genet. 2012 Jul; 29(7): 631–635. doi: 10.1007/s10815-012-9760-8

80. Sabna Kotta, Shahid H. Ansari,and Javed Ali. Exploring scientifically proven herbal aphrodisiacs. Pharmacogn Rev. 2013 Jan-Jun; 7(13): 1–10. doi: 10.4103/0973-7847.112832. https://www.ncbi.nlm.nih.gov/pmc/articles/PMC3731873/

81. Kenjale R, Shah R, Sathaye S. Effects of Chlorophytum borivilianum on sexual behaviour and sperm count in male rats. Phytother Res. 2008 Jun; 22(6):796-801.

82. Lampiao F, Krom D, du Plessis SS. The in vitro effects of Mondia whitei on human sperm motility parameters. Phytother Res. 2008;22:1272–3

83. Safarinejad MR, Shafiei N, Safarinejad S. An open label, randomized, fixed-dose, crossover study comparing efficacy and safety of sildenafil citrate and saffron (Crocus sativus Linn.) for treating erectile dysfunction in men naïve to treatment. Int J Impot Res. 2010;22:240–50

84. Tajuddin SA, Shamshad A, Abdul L, Iqbal A. Aphrodisiac activity of 50% ethanolic extracts of Myristica fragrans Houtt. (nutmeg) and Syzygium aromaticum (L) Merr. and Perry (clove) in male mice: A comparative study. Complement Altern Med. 2003;3:6

85. Bahmanpour S, Talaei T, Vojdani Z, Panjehshahin MR, Poostpasand A, Zareei S. Effect of Phoenix dactylifera pollen on sperm parameters and reproductive system of adult male rats. Iran J Med Sci. 2006;31(4):208–212

86. Cicero AF, Bandieri E, Arletti R. Lepidium meyenii Walp. improves sexual behaviour in male rats independently from its action on spontaneous locomotor activity. J Ethnopharmacol. 2001;75:225–9

87. Chen X. Cardiovascular protection by ginsenosides and their nitric oxide releasing action. Clin Exp Pharmacol Physiol. 1996;23:728–32

88. Adeniyi AA, Brindley GS, Pryor JP, Ralph DJ. Yohimbine in the treatment of orgasmic dysfunction. Asian J Androl. 2007;9:403–7

89. Yakubu MT, Akanji MA, Oladiji AT. Effects of oral administration of aqueous extract of Fadogia agrestis (Schweinf. Ex Hiern) stem on some testicular function indices of male rats. J Ethnopharmacol. 2008;115:288–

90. Ratnasooriya WD, Dharmasiri MG. Effects of Terminalia catappa seeds on sexual behaviour and fertility of male rats. Asian J Androl. 2000;2:213–9.

91. Patel DK, Kumar R, Prasad SK, Hemalatha S. Pharmacologically screened aphrodisiac plant: A review of current scientific literature. Asian Pac J Trop Biomed. 2011;1:S131–8.

Ali ST, Rakkah NI. Probable neuro sexual mode of action of Casimiroa edulis seed extract versus correction of verses sildenafil citrate (Viagra (tm)) on mating behavior in normal male rats. Pak J Pharm Sci. 2008;21:1–6.

92. Estrada-Reyes R, Ortiz-López P, Gutiérrez-Ortíz J, Martínez-Mota L. Turnera diffusa Wild (Turneraceae) recovers sexual behavior in sexually exhausted males. J Ethnopharmacol. 2009;123:423–9

93. Pallav Sengupta et al. Role of Withania somnifera (Ashwagandha) in the management of male infertility. https://doi.org/10.1016/j.rbmo.2017.11.007. https://www.rbmojournal.com/article/S1472-6483(17)30625-9/pdf

94. Carlo Bulletti et al. Endometriosis and infertility. J Assist Reprod Genet. 2010 Aug; 27(8): 441–447. Published online 2010 Jun 25. doi: 10.1007/s10815-010-9436-1. Endometriosis and infertility.

95. Swati Dongre, Deepak Langade, and Sauvik Bhattacharyya. Efficacy and Safety of Ashwagandha (Withania somnifera) Root Extract in Improving Sexual Function in Women: A Pilot Study. Biomed Res Int. 2015; 2015: 284154.

96. Sally Lewis. 50 Things you can do today to increase your fertility. Summerdale Publisher 2011